Psychology for Social Workers

Social work education has undergone major changes, with anti-discriminatory practice being a high-priority area in professional training. *Psychology for Social Workers* provides an introductory text which will help qualifying and practising social workers to:

- understand and counteract the impact of discrimination;
- work in an ethnically sensitive way;
- demonstrate an awareness of ways to combat both individual and institutional racism through anti-racist practice.

Drawing together research material and literature on black perspectives in human development and behaviour from North America and Britain, it provides a starting point that will inspire discussion and debate in the social work field and will generate future theoretical and research questions. Among the topics covered are black perspectives in group work and the family, identity development and academic achievement in black children, and mental health issues in relation to black people.

Updated throughout to cover recent developments in the field, this second edition is an essential introductory text for all social workers in training and practice and for their teachers and trainers.

Lena Robinson is Professor of Social Work at the University of the West of Scotland, UK.

D0218039

Psychology for Social Workers

Black perspectives on human development and behaviour

Lena Robinson

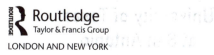

LONDON AND NEW YORK

First published 1995
by Routledge

This edition published 2009
by Routledge
2 Park Square, Milton Park, Abingdon, Oxon OX14 4RN

Simultaneously published in the USA and Canada
by Routledge
270 Madison Avenue, New York, NY 10016

Routledge is an imprint of the Taylor & Francis Group, an informa business

© 2009 Lena Robinson

Typeset in Sabon by Pindar NZ, Auckland, New Zealand
Printed and bound in Great Britain by CPI Antony Rowe,
Chippenham, Wiltshire

British Library Cataloguing in Publication Data
A catalogue record for this book is available from the British Library

Library of Congress Cataloging-in-Publication Data
Robinson, Lena, 1957-
  Psychology for social workers: Black perspectives on human
development and behaviour/Lena Robinson. — 2nd ed.
    p. cm.
  Includes bibliographical references.
  1. Blacks—Services for—Great Britain. 2. Social work with
minorities—Great Britain. 3. Social service and race relations—Great
Britain. 4. Social service—Great Britain—Psychological aspects. 5.
Race awareness—Great Britain. I. Title.
  HV3199.B52G77 2009
  362.84'96041—dc22   2008029444

ISBN 10: 0-415-36912-6 (hbk)
ISBN 10: 0-415-36913-4 (pbk)

ISBN 13: 978-0-415-36912-1 (hbk)
ISBN 13: 978-0-415-36913-8 (pbk)

Contents

Introduction

During the late 1980s, social work education in Britain 'became increasingly aware of the impact of oppression and discrimination on clients and communities' (Thompson, 2001: 1). For example, the Central Council for the Education and Training of Social Workers (CCETSW) requirements for the Diploma in Social Work award attached a high priority to an anti-discriminatory approach in college and placement teaching and assessment. (see Central Council for Education and Training in Social Work Paper 30, 1991a).

However, CCETSW's anti-racist initiative 'came under scrutiny and hostility from a range of groups [including] the media, government and from inside the [social work] profession itself' (Penketh, 2000: 123). But, recent evidence of institutional racism, e.g. the Stephen Lawrence Inquiry (Macpherson, 1999), highlights the need for a commitment to anti-racist practice (Penketh, 2000). The Race Relations (Amendment) Act 2000 was introduced as an effort to combat institutional racism. The Act:

> requires named public authorities to review their policies and procedures; to remove discrimination and the possibility of discrimination; and to actively promote race equality'. Anti-racist social work 'opened attention to other forms of discrimination, and contributed to anti-discriminatory practice becoming part of the fabric of social work education and practice
>
> (Graham, 2007: 3)

The term 'black' in this book has been used to describe people from South Asian, African and Caribbean backgrounds. While it is necessary to emphasize the heterogeneity of black people, of equal importance is the consideration of how black people in Britain differ from the white group. The three main areas in which the experience of black people in this country has been distinct from that of the white group are: racism and discrimination; the history of colonialism and imperialism; and 'the existence of immigration and nationality legislation that has historically been instituted to keep out [black people]' (Singh, 1992: 31). As Hall comments:

> 'black' was coined as a way of referencing the common experience of racism and marginalisation in Britain and came to provide the organising category of a new politics of resistance, amongst groups and communities with, in fact, very different histories, traditions and ethnic identities.
>
> (Hall, 1992: 252)

In Britain, 'Asian groups claim they are not "black" as part of their struggle to assert their own particularity in historical, cultural, ethical and lingustic terms' (Dominelli, 1997: 7). This book does not use the term 'black' to deny the uniqueness of different ethnic groups. It is used 'as an inclusive political term to counter the divisive aspects of racism' (Dominelli, 1997: 7). Campbell and Rose stress that 'Although black means solidarity in the face of oppression, it does not exclude diversity of culture, religion, language, origin, etc.' (Campbell and Rose, 1992: 17).

After completing this book some readers will wish for more comparisons between African Caribbeans and South Asians. It was never my intent to provide a detailed comparison, and it is clearly beyond the scope of this book. However, there is a need for more literature and research exploring the critical differences between ethnic groups.

This book attempts to articulate, from a black perspective, a framework for social work practice that applies to black people in general. The main aim of the book is to identify a number of practice principles applicable to all black people, rather than delineating specific principles for each major black group. The framework for developing a black perspective is based on the notion of common experiences that black people in Britain share.

A black perspective in psychology (see Chapter 1) is committed to replacing the white distortion of black reality with black writings of black experience. It is about valuing differences and recognizing strengths. Social work education and training in Britain is under the control of white educators and practitioners, who have failed to address satisfactorily the issue of racism in either social work theory or practice (Dominelli, 1997). As mainstream social work policies and practices are fundamentally Eurocentric, social work needs to get rid of its Eurocentrism in order to become anti-racist. Social work education cannot allow the Eurocentric perspective to dominate social work training. What is currently obvious is that the black perspective can no longer be a peripheral subject in social work education and training. It is a central requirement of social work training. This book attempts to examine issues which are considered central to the development of a black perspective in the teaching of psychological theory on social work courses. The General Social Care Council (GSCC) played an important role in the introduction of the new social work degree in 2003. It has 'the responsibility for the approval of social work courses under Section 63 of the Care Standards Act 2000' (DoH, 2002: 1). The requirements for the new degree in social work state that 'all students need to undertake specific learning and assessment in human growth and development' (DoH, 2002: 3). Although the document does not state that these theories are psychological or derived from psychology, it is obvious that psychology has an important contribution to make towards an understanding of human behaviour. Explanations of black behaviour which are alternative to white perspectives are developed here.

The subject disciplines in social work education are based on Anglocentric models which take white British culture, history and achievements as the norm. Social work has turned to the social sciences, particularly psychology, for accounts of human behaviour which can be applied in practice. Psychological theory and human development are considered largely in terms of the white British middle-class standard. For example, discussions about the family centre on the white middle-class nuclear family as the favoured type. Variations from this are considered 'deviant' and consequently undesirable (Segal, 1983; Lorde, 1984; Bernard, 2001; Robinson, 2007).

British social work operates within the framework of middle-class values. Social workers are mostly white middle-class people who are very much removed from the black population. My aim in writing this book for social workers is to provide them with the knowledge base to carry out psychologically informed social work from a black perspective. Little of the current psychological literature in Britain (both general and specifically for social workers) has been approached from an articulated theory-based black perspective. The main psychology texts (for example, Nicolson, Bayne and Owen (2006) *Applied Psychology for Social Workers*) written for social work students take little or no account of the black perspective. In the social work literature one finds racial stereotypes of: Asian women as passive and sexually repressed (Khan, 1979); Asian girls as 'caught between two cultures'

(Anwar, 1998; Triseliotis, 1972); and African Caribbean families as unable to provide the environment in which the nuclear family prospers (Bernard, 2001; Fitzherbert, 1967). By presenting black people in this light, these authors endorse the implicit assumption that (white) British institutions and culture are superior.

Some authors have argued that child development research often lacks a black perspective and, where research exists, its validity has been questioned because of its possible distortion by researchers with Eurocentric approaches (for example, White, 2004; Wilson, 1981). White (1980, 2004) maintains that traditional psychology's use of an Anglo middle-class frame of reference gives it a distorted view of the adaptive ability of black children and the black family.

Mainstream child psychology does not usually consider race and race awareness as an important variable on the child's mental, emotional and personality development. According to Wilson:

> the shape of the black child's intellect and personality is determined by the concept of race, race awareness and race politics – and psychology which fails to treat these items as major personality and mental variables is not adequate to deal with the black child. This has been the greatest failure of American developmental, educational and clinical psychology.
>
> (Wilson, 1978: 8)

Child psychology is central to the learning needs of social workers. Social work courses in Britain need to consider black child studies as a unique and important area of specialization. Studies have found a disproportionate number of black children in care (Barn *et al.*, 1997; Ahmed, 2005).

This book aims to provide a basic introduction to psychological knowledge – from a black perspective – for social work students and practitioners. It argues that social workers need to take the black perspective seriously if they are going to find ways of improving their practice. The black perspective should not simply be 'tacked on' as an afterthought. These ideas must be integral to social work education. Traditional principles and theories in psychology have not had sufficient explanatory power to account for the behaviour of black people in Britain.

Black psychologists (mainly in the USA) have, therefore, presented alternative perspectives on black child development, black families, black education, black mental health and personality development. Most of the psychological research on black children and black families has concentrated on African-American families. It may be some time before such perspectives are developed and articulated in Britain by psychologists and social workers. In the meantime, some understanding of current research and theory is needed to guide present understanding, action and research in Britain. Social work training must question whether theories which have originated in Euro-American settings have relevance in working with black clients in Britain. As mainstream social work policies and practices are fundamentally Eurocentric, social work needs to get rid of its Eurocentrism in order to become anti-racist.

This book draws together research material and literature on black perspectives in human development and behaviour from North America and the United Kingdom. However, there are limitations to the extent and depth an introductory text can cover. I prefer to cover some topics in relative depth, rather than write a catalogue. There is definitely a need to develop a black perspective in psychology. This book has been revised to take account of the latest developments in this field. It is my hope that this book is a starting point that will inspire discussion and debate in the social work field, and will generate theoretical and research questions for years to come.

Chapter 1 discusses the emergence of a black perspective in psychology, and attempts to explore the issue of why a psychological perspective specific to black people is necessary. It argues that traditional principles and theories have not had sufficient explanatory power to account for the behaviour of blacks. This edition includes a section on cross-cultural psychology. Black psychology has become part of ethnic or cross-cultural psychology in recent years. Chapter 2 focuses on impression formation as it relates to black people. There is a section in this edition on differences in communication styles between high and low context cultures. Differences between cultures in the perception of time are also explored. Chapter 3 attempts to develop a black perspective in group work. Chapter 4 discusses issues relevant to the black family in Britain. Particular attention is given to the existing pathology-oriented black family literature. This edition includes a section on racial socialization. It is argued that racial socialization is relevant to understanding the socialization practices of black families. Chapter 5 contains a discussion of identity development in black children. It draws on the work of several black psychologists who are at the forefront of identity development research relative to black people. There is a section on acculturation theory in this edition. Acculturation models are concerned with the extent to which ethnic identity is maintained when an ethnic group is in continuous contact with the dominant group. Issues related to identity formation among mixed parentage children and adolescents are also discussed in this edition.

Chapter 6 presents a discussion of the factors that influence the academic achievement of black children. Chapter 7 focuses on mental health issues as they relate to black people. Recent developments in this area are included in this edition.

1 The black perspective in psychology

In this chapter I will review the origin and development of a black perspective in psychology, with a discussion of why this perspective is necessary, and its implications for social work training. I will argue that traditional psychological theories have not had sufficient explanatory power to account for the behaviour of black people.

This chapter draws upon the valuable discussions of various black authors: Jackson (1979), White (1972, 1984, 2004), Baldwin (1976, 1980) Kambon (2004), none of which are readily available in traditional psychology. It will also highlight recent developments. In recent years black psychology has become part of a larger movement in psychology – cross-cultural psychology (Belgrave and Allison, 2005; Jones, 2004).

Inadequacies of Western psychology

Psychology is regarded as 'the science of human behaviour'. This definition implies that 'human behaviour in all parts of the world must be investigated, not just those aspects of behaviour conveniently available to investigators in highly industrialized nations with a history of scientific endeavor' (Triandis and Brislin, 1984: 1006). The exclusive limitation of psychology's databases to research in Western populations is responsible for certain inadequacies in current psychological theories and literature. For example, Curran pointed out that developmental psychology texts are generally 'based on the behaviour of Western children in very contrived situations which bear little relation to those children's familiar environments' (Curran, 1984: 2).

White psychologists have maintained that they were objective scientists whose research findings were politically neutral. Yet, they have embraced a number of racist themes in describing, explaining, and modifying black behaviour. These themes can be seen in conceptions of black people's abilities and personality, in suggestions for the education of blacks, and in suggestions for work with blacks in counselling and psychotherapy.

Hayes argues that 'psychology adopted a definition of science that would allow [its] inclusion among the scientific disciplines' (Hayes, 1980: 37). Furthermore, psychology 'adopted rules of science which would allow psychologists to find expression for their cultural and racial biases while presenting themselves as scientific investigators of human behaviour' (Hayes, 1980: 37). Other writers (for example, Guthrie, 2004; Longino, 1990; Onwubu, 1990) have indicated that social science research is influenced by ideology and cultural values.

Many psychologists, both black and white, have noted the inadequacies of Western psychology. These reviews (Akbar, 1981; Asante, 1980; Baldwin, 1976; Clark, 1972; Guthrie, 2004; Jackson, 1979; Kambon, 2004; Nobles, 1973, 2004; White, 2004) have in general suggested that the failure of Western psychology is found in both its approach to and conception of the study of people. Western psychology's attempt at establishing a normative standard for human cognition, emotion and behaviour is questionable.

> Eurocentric-oriented research has tended to develop paradigms to interpret different scoring patterns that African-Americans consistently exhibit relative to European-Americans on so-called measures of self-concept/self-esteem, personal motivation and attributions, ability and achievement, etc., as reflecting psychosocial deficit and pathology (Baldwin, 1976, 1979). Invariably, then, the major conclusion drawn from this approach is that African-Americans are culturally disadvantaged or deprived relative to European-Americans.
>
> (Baldwin and Hopkins, 1990: 40)

Psychological theories of personality, intelligence, motivation, learning, language development, self-concept, etc., were standardized on whites and applied to black people. A model of white middle-class personality has been 'utilized as a measuring stick against which all other psychological development is assessed' (Sinha, 1983: 7); 'the standard against which others must measure up' (Segall *et al.*, 1990: 93).

Most psychologists would agree that Jean Piaget, a Swiss psychologist, was the most influential developmental psychologist of the twentieth century. He identified a number of distinct stages of intellectual development, and proposed that the child moved through each of these stages in turn. The four main stages are: sensori-motor; pre-operational;

concrete operational; and formal operational. In each of the stages the child is able to tackle different kinds of problems successfully (see Piaget, 1970, for a detailed account of his theory of cognitive development). If we examine his work on cognitive development, it becomes clear that the skills Piaget selected to study the mind are particularly well suited to Western technological culture. Joseph *et al.* address this issue:

> If one assumes, as Piagetians do for example, that there is a 'natural' sequence of development which is universal, with a 'natural' fixed end-point (the attainment of formal reasoning) and that these stages are 'naturally' attained (not through social tutoring) and that this is the path development will take unless there is something lacking in the environment, then the interpretation that some non-western cultures may not be competent at formal reasoning may indeed be seen as ethnocentric.
>
> (Joseph *et al.*, 1990: 12–13)

Cole *et al.* argue that 'cultural differences in cognition reside more in the situations to which particular cognitive processes are applied than in the existence of a process in one cultural group and its absence in another' (1971: 233).

The conventionally accepted paradigms and discoveries of Western psychology do not provide an understanding of black people. Even a casual observation of the history of psychology will demonstrate that psychological literature from the last 100 years has been based on observations primarily of Europeans, predominantly male and over-whelmingly middle-class. General psychology has failed to provide a full and accurate understanding of black reality. In fact, its utilization has, in many instances, resulted in the pathologization of black people (Jones, 2004).

Guthrie, in his book *Even the Rat was White* (1976), provides us with an overview of the problems and inadequacies of Western psychology. For example, in regard to psychology and race, Guthrie points out that Western psychologists not only provided inaccurate data that led to racist conclusions, but that their behaviour and conduct also called into question the intentions of psychological research. This latter point is important. Has the covert and, in some instances, overt 'intention' of Western psychology been to accept as true the inferiority of black people? Guthrie argues that, in regard to African people, Western psychology in general accepted, as a basic a priori assumption, that African people were inferior.

Those thinkers who have shaped the thought of Euro-American

psychology have all directly or indirectly asserted the superiority of European races over non-European races. Despite the diversity of the various schools of Western psychology, they seem to merge unequivocally in their assumption of the Eurocentric point of view and the superiority of people of European descent. It is not surprising, therefore, that the conclusions reached from the application of their concepts and methods are invariably of the inferiority of non-European peoples.

In 1869, Francis Galton published his major work on *Hereditary Genius* and argued that, based on his 'scientific scale of racial values', he was able to conclude that the average intellectual standard of the Negro was at least two grades below that of whites. He proposed that a new science should start up, called eugenics, by which intelligent individuals would have children together and less intelligent people would be prevented from having children, through compulsory sterilization, in an attempt to improve the quality of the human race.

Edward Thorndike, who was thought by many to be America's greatest psychologist, wrote, in his book *Human Nature and the Social Order*, that 'The principle of eliminating bad genes is so thoroughly sound that almost any practice based on it is likely to do more good than harm' (1940: 44). Thorndike, who also helped to develop the army intelligence test in the USA, believed and stated 'that the institution of slavery existed because the black man's original nature was conducive to exploitation' (Thorndike, 1940).

In furthering Western psychology's understanding of black people, Lewis Terman (1916) noted that Afro-American and other ethnic minority children:

> are uneducable beyond the nearest rudiments of training. No amount of school instruction will ever make them intelligent voters or capable citizens in the true sense of the word ... their dullness seems to be racial, or at least inherent in the family stock from which they come ... children of this group should be segregated in special classes and be given instruction which is concrete and practical. They cannot master abstractions, but they can often be made efficient workers. There is no possibility at present of convincing society that they should not be allowed to reproduce, although from a eugenic point of view they constitute a grave problem because of their unusual prolific breeding.
>
> (Terman, 1916: 91–2)

William McDougall, who has been called the 'Father of Social Psychology', also advanced the position that all people of African descent were innately intellectually inferior to whites (McDougall, 1921). In addition, he promoted the dogma of instincts in people: for example, that inborn and unlearned response tendencies determined social behaviour. The widespread stereotyping of black people as easy-going, happy and lazy resulted from this concept (Guthrie, 1976).

Social work practice in Britain and the USA has been influenced greatly by the psychoanalytic approach (for discussion, see Yelloly, 1980, 1990). This approach is based on Sigmund Freud's work, but has been developed by neo-Freudians (for example, Erikson, Melanie Klein, and Jung). In his book *Totem and Taboo* Sigmund Freud (1912–13) refers to the practices and behaviours of African peoples as 'savage' or 'primitive'. Carl Jung (at one time Freud's star pupil) has been re-ferred to as the father of 'transpersonal psychology'. He believed that certain psychological disorders found among Americans were due to the presence of black people in America. He noted that 'The causes for the American energetic sexual repression can be found in the spe-cific American complex, namely to living together with "lower races, especially with Negroes"' (Jung, 1950: 29). Dalal (1988) maintains that Jung considered black people to be inferior and not just differ-ent. However, he says that 'it would be a mistake to assume that in the field of psychotherapy the charge of racism can only be levelled at Jung and his theories' (Dalal, 1988: 21). He chose to focus on Jung, however, because of 'his popularity, and because his racism is invisible to modern Jungians' (Dalal, 1988: 21). It is important to note that psychometric projective techniques such as the Rorschach Ink Blot Test (Rorschach, 1942) and Thematic Apperception Test (Murray, 1938) depend heavily upon psychoanalytical theoretical underpinnings for their interpretations.

Baldwin (1976) observed that the standards of observation which have led to persistent conclusions of the 'social pathology' of black behaviour resulted from the Eurocentric assumptions in the use of measures of black behaviour.

> The traditional social pathology view of black behaviours is there-fore based on a European conception or definition of reality, or more precisely, a European distortion of the reality of black people. Its rise to prominence in the psychological literature, naturally then, merely reflects the vested social power of Euro-American psychology (and white people generally in European American culture) to legitimate European definitions of reality rather than the necessary objective credibility appeal of its presumed validity.
>
> (Baldwin, 1976: 8)

A main feature of Eurocentric psychology is the assumption among psychologists that people are alike in all important respects. In order to explain 'universal human phenomena', white psychologists established a normative standard of behaviour against which all other cultural groups were to be measured. What appeared as normal or abnormal was always in comparison to how closely a specific thought or behaviour corresponded to that of white people. Hence, normality is established on a model of the middle-class, Caucasian male of European descent. The more one approximates this model in appearance, values and behaviour, the more 'normal' one is considered to be. The obvious advantage for Europeans (whites) is that such norms confirm their reality as the reality, and flaunt statements of their supremacy as scientifically based 'fact'. The major problem with such normative assumptions for non-European people is the inevitable conclusion of deviance on the part of anyone unlike this model. In fact, the more distinct or distant you are from this model, the more pathological you are considered to be.

For many white psychologists, the word 'different' when applied to black people became synonymous with 'deficient', rather than simply different. For example, many psychological tests (standardized on white people), are inappropriately applied to blacks, causing them to appear less intelligent or deficient. Guthrie (1976) has discussed the problems of culturally biased psychologists who administer and interpret culturally biased psychological tests.

White asserts that 'it is difficult if not impossible to understand the lifestyles of black people using traditional psychological theories, developed by white psychologists to explain white behaviour' (White, 1972: 5). White goes on to state that, when these theories are applied to black people, many weakness-dominated and inferiority-oriented conclusions are discovered. An analysis of the psychological literature on black people will illustrate White's point.

An example which White offers is of the designation of 'culturally deprived' to a group of black youngsters whom he describes as having developed the kind of 'mental toughness and survival skills, in terms of coping with life, which make them in many ways superior to their white age-mates'. He continues: 'these black youngsters know how to deal effectively with bill collectors ... they recognize very early that they exist in an environment which is sometimes both complicated and hostile' (White, 1972: 6).

Models of Western psychological research on black people

Various models can be traced in the Western (Eurocentric) psychological research of black and minority groups (Sue, 1978, 2006; Thomas and Sillen, 1972). These models include: the inferiority model; the deficit (deprivations) model; and the multi-cultural model.

The inferiority model maintains that blacks are intellectually, physically, and mentally inferior to whites – due to genetics/heredity. It focuses on the role of genes in explaining differences between blacks and whites. The model apparently gave some authors a scientific basis for regarding blacks as inferior (Jensen, 1969, 1987; Rushton, 1988a, 1988b). Rushton has proposed a theory in sociobiology whereby Asians, Caucasians, and Africans, as a result of evolution, may be hierarchically ranked such that Mongoloids > Caucasoids > Negroids. Fairchild, in an article entitled 'Scientific racism: the cloak of objectivity' (1991), challenges Rushton's conclusions. He argues that 'Rushton's sociobiology of racial differences is unscientific in its assumptions and interpretations, and therefore may properly be regarded as scientific racism' (Fairchild, 1991: 112).

The deficit/deficiency model contends that blacks are deficient with respect to intelligence, cognitive styles, and family structure – due to lack of proper environmental stimulation, racism, and oppressive conditions. From this deficit model came such hypo-theses as 'cultural deprivation', which presumed that, due to inadequate exposure to Eurocentric values, norms, customs, and lifestyles, blacks were 'culturally deprived' and required cultural enrichment. Implicit in the concept of cultural deprivation, however, is the notion that the dominant white middle-class culture established the normative standard. Thus, any behaviours, values, and lifestyles that differed from the Euro-American norm were seen as deficient.

The multicultural model states that all culturally distinct groups have strengths and limitations. The differences between ethnic groups are viewed as simply different – rather than being viewed as deficient. This model has helped researchers to focus on culture-specific models in a multicultural context (for example, Sue and Wagner, 1973; Sue, 1981 – in regard to Asian Americans). Minority groups took the initiative in defining themselves rather than being defined by the deficit/deficiency models of the white culture.

Only a few white psychologists (for example, Jensen, 1969) accept the idea that black people are at birth genetically inferior to whites in intellectual potential. Most psychologists take the view:

that black people are culturally deprived and psychologically mal-adjusted because the environment in which they were reared as children and in which they continue to rear their own children lacks the necessary early experiences to prepare them for, generally speaking, achievement within an Anglo middle-class frame of reference.

(White, 1980: 5)

We can see that implicit in the concept of cultural deprivation is the belief that the normative standard is the white middle-class culture. Therefore, any behaviour that is different from the white norm is labelled as deficient.

The tradition of viewing black people as deviants from the 'norm' is reflected in research on the black family. Black families have been studied using Eurocentric frameworks. For example, based on the Eurocentric norm and models of Freudian psychology, Moynihan (1965) concluded that the 'Black family' was essentially pathogenic and responsible for the origin of many psychological and social problems of African Americans. He wrote: 'At the heart of the deterioration of the fabric of Negro society is the deterioration of the Negro family .... It is the fundamental source of the weakness of the Negro Community at present' (Moynihan, 1965: 15).

Moynihan labelled the black family a 'tangle of pathology'. In his analysis he regarded the black woman as maintaining a matriarchal culture. In turn, the black matriarchy model was viewed as maintaining pathology because it did not conform to the 'normal' family structures of the white culture (Moynihan, 1965).

A number of writers (Belgrave and Allison, 2006; Billingsley, 1968; Nobles, 1978; McAdoo, 1981a, 1981b) have challenged the deficit views of black family life, in which positive psychological factors have been ignored, while the 'pathological' factors have been heightened. Other researchers have advanced more positive views of the black family and have examined the strengths in black families (McAdoo, 1981a, 1981b; McAdoo and McAdoo, 1985). These issues will be discussed in Chapter 4.

The social work literature has done much to reproduce the myths and distortions about the black family. As Stubbs states, 'Despite some later recognition of the strengths of black family structures, most of the literature continues to emphasise cultural pathology as an explanation for the problems of black families' (1988: 99).

Another example of the tradition of viewing black people as deviants from the 'norm' is reflected in research on the black child. Many researchers (for example, Moynihan, 1965; Jensen, 1969; Deutsch, 1968; Bernstein, 1961; Hunt, 1961) maintain that the black child:

> (a) is delinquent because he has a defective superego, (b) is emotionally disturbed because he refuses to adjust and upsets existing settings, (c) scores differently on IQ tests than whites because he has inferior genes, (d) lives in a ghetto because he comes from a deficient family with dominant mothers and pregnant sisters, (e) fails to obtain jobs and promotions because he lacks proper work habits and a 'competent self', (f) fails in school because he is 'culturally deprived', and (g) fails in virtually all aspects of life because he forever carries the scars of oppression obtained at home during preschool years.
>
> (Gordon, 1973: 91)

Many psychologists and social workers assume that the black child is a white child who 'happens' to be painted black. This implies that the social, emotional, mental, and physical developmental patterns of the white middle-class child have become the optimal standard by which the black child is measured. Wilson (1981, 1992) argues that there are critical differences between black and white children, and psychologists have failed to consider the study of the black child as an important area of specialization. Consequently, our understanding of the psychological development of the child is based on research on white children by white psychologists. In American and British psychological literature the black child is treated as an afterthought, as a contrast to the white child, never as a subject matter in its own right.

Psychological research has often been used to support racist ideas and practices in American and British society. The theories, methodologies, findings, and conclusions generated by white psychologists have been used to try to demonstrate that blacks and other racial minorities are mentally inferior to whites. There exists a wealth of data that indicate that the psychometric tools used in psychology are not only biased against black people, but fall short of providing any useful data in predicting talents, capabilities, or skills of the majority of black children. The black child is being judged by a test which is based on an experience which he/she has not been allowed to have, and which gives no credibility to his/her experiences. In most standardized tests, subtests are heavily loaded with content from the white middle-class culture. Therefore, it should not be surprising that individuals from that group do better on such tests than individuals from black groups. Therefore, for black groups these tests measure only their familiarity with white culture.

Research carried out by Williams (1981) demonstrated that, when a test is based on a black group's perspective and experiences, they will do better on the test than the white group. His research on the Black Intelligence Test of Cultural Homogeneity (BITCH), which is a black, culture-specific test, shows that blacks score consistently higher than whites on this test, which is based on black culture. The test, consisting of 100 culturally biased items, was administered to samples of African-American and European-American high-school students and adults in the United States. The results consistently showed significantly different scoring patterns between these two groups, with the African Americans scoring at least thirty points higher than European Americans. This illustrates that, if a test is made specifically for a particular group (as most standardized tests are made for the white middle class), then one would expect members of that group to score higher on the test than members from outgroups. Although there is much doubt regarding the validity of intelligence tests, psychologists have used and continue to use them as valid (Williams *et al.*, 2004).

The above examples were used to illustrate the need for a psychological explanation and analysis of black lifestyles, which emerges from the framework of the black experience.

Due to the negative images of black people that have emerged from the Eurocentric approaches, it is clear that it is imperative to apply an alternative frame of reference. It can be seen that traditional psychology has failed to provide an accurate understanding of the black reality. In fact, its use has, in many instances, resulted in the pathologization of black people (Jones, 2004).

Toward a black perspective in psychology

There is a consensus among most black psychologists and professionals that explanations of black behaviour which are alternative to white European perspectives must be developed.

A black perspective in psychology is concerned with combating (negative) racist and stereotypic, weakness-dominated and inferiority-oriented conclusions about black people. This perspective is interested in the psychological well-being of black people and is critical of research paradigms and theoretical formulations that have a potentially oppressive effect on black people. White psychology has offered deficit-oriented psychological explanations about the behaviour of black people. These deficit theories have been used to explain much of the behaviour of blacks as individuals and as a group.

The black perspective is critical of the white middle-class norm in psychology – and argues that it is necessary to analyse black behaviour in the context of its own norms. Much of the work and research involved in developing a black perspective in psychology was initiated in the USA by black psychologists.

In the USA, the development of a black perspective has advanced through two overlapping phases. The first phase questioned the conclusions of white psychologists whose research and theories inevitably specified some deficit, deficiency, and/or distortion in the psychological make-up of black people as compared to whites. The second phase questioned the assumptions upon which white psychologists based their theories and research, while indicating that their biased results were partially a function of these assumptions. A black perspective must be concerned with developing new theories and psychological tests which are applicable to black people. Smith argues that psychological innovations 'are needed to aid in deriving truth about black behaviour; they are needed to combat racism; [and] to aid Blacks in dealing more effectively with black communities' (Smith, 1979: 11).

In the USA the efforts of black psychologists have been felt in the areas of community mental health, education, intelligence and ability testing, professional training, forensic psychology, and criminal justice. Some of the goals of the Association of Black Psychologists, which was formed in 1968 in the USA, are: to improve the psychological well-being of black people in America; to promote an understanding of black people through positive approaches to research; to develop an approach to psychology that is consistent with the experience of black people; and to define mental health in accordance with newly established psychological concepts and standards regarding black people. Since its establishment the Association has played an important role in stimulating and contributing to the body of literature available on black people.

The black perspective in Britain has referred to the knowledge base of black research in the USA, and adapted it to fit in with the British experience. The development of a black psychology is more advanced in the USA than in Britain. It would appear that in Britain only a few social scientists acknowledge the failure of general psychology to provide an accurate understanding of black reality and the pathologization of black people resulting from applications of Eurocentric norms. More research from a black perspective needs to be carried out in the areas of mental health, education, intelligence and ability, personality, motivation, learning, language development, the family, and self-concept.

Not only will the understanding of the black frame of reference enable social workers to come up with more accurate and comprehensive explanations, but it will also enable them to build the kind of programmes within the black world which capitalize on the strengths of black people. A strengths-coping perspective tends to describe black behaviour almost exclusively as positive adaptations and does not attempt to utilize a white cultural framework as a standard for all behavioural phenomena. Such a perspective is illustrated in Hill's (1972, 2003, 1998) model of black families, which cites kinship bonds, religiosity, and achievement orientation as examples of some strengths indigenous to black families (see Chapter 4).

Issues in developing a black perspective in psychology

Most black psychologists appear to recognize basic problems in the applicability of Western (white-European) psychology to the experiences of black or African people. Black psychologists have felt for a long time that the description of black behaviour as deviant, abnormal, and pathological was inaccurate. Because of the racism inherent in traditional Western psychological models, black psychologists felt a need to branch out and develop a discipline that would be more applicable to the description and explanation of black life. It was in the context of a 'paradigm of racism' that black psychology was formally conceived. Thus, black psychology was a reaction. Black psychology is self-affirmative, particularly in its denial of the denigrating conceptualizations of European-American psychology (Akbar, 2004). European American concepts 'are appropriate for a time and a context, i.e., the time and context that views the African American [black person] as a deviant from the anglo world for those observers who maintain the insignificance of race and cultural plurality may still find such an approach appropriate and valuable' (Akbar, 2004: 37). Black psychology 'represents an effort to come to grips with the overwhelming ethnocentrism of European American psychology with a counter-ethnocentrism (Akbar, 2004: 38). A recent update to White's (1970) article entitled 'Toward a Black Psychology' in Jones (2004) strongly advocates a Black psychology defined by black people.

There are diverse views among black psychologists on the development of a black psychological perspective. Many black psychologists, while accepting the need for a black psychology, do not view it as an independent activity separate from Western psychology (for example, Cross, 1971; Guthrie, 1976; White, 1972; Comer and Pouissant, 1992).

Comer and Poussaint (1992) argue that there is no distinct black psychology or white psychology. However, they acknowledge that psychological practices in the USA have been white-dominated and are often culturally biased and racist. White (1972, 2004) maintains that not all traditional white psychological theory is useless, and that it was the duty of psychologists to incorporate what is useful into black psychology and reject the rest. An example of a useful theory is found in the views of the existential psychologists. Their theory applies to the lives of black people, because they take the view that, in order to understand what a person is and the way he/she views the world, one must have some awareness of his/her experiential background, especially as it might include experiences with the institutions such as the home, family, and the immediate neighbourhood which directly affect the person's life.

Other black psychologists argue that black psychology is independent from Western psychology because 'African (Black) psychology ... derives naturally from the "worldview" or philosophical premises underlying African culture (as does Western psychology relative to the worldview of European culture' (Baldwin, 1991: 126).

For some African-American psychologists (White, 1972; Pugh, 1972) the term black psychology refers to 'an accurate workable theory of black behaviour drawn from the authentic experience of black people in American society' (Baldwin, 1991: 126). For Louis Williams:

> Black psychology is the psychological consequence of being black. In this work, problems and issues of psychology have been presented from a variety of operational viewpoints, including those of Eastern, African, Western, and Afro-American experience. [This approach] ... centers on a general principle of the uniqueness of the black experience .... [Therefore] out of the authentic experience of black people we must build a viable psychology ... this notion is central in the definition of Black psychology.
>
> (Williams, 1978: 3)

Guthrie (2004) maintains that 'black psychology is an outgrowth of "Third World" philosophies which are not committed to the authenticity of traditional European and American psychology, but are born out of a need promulgated through neglect rather than traditional theoretical stances' (Guthrie, 2004: 48). Guthrie (2004) envisions black psychology as a scientific study of behaviour attempting to understand life as it is lived. Nobles (2004: 58) considers a rationale for black psychology as: 'engaging in a critique and rejection of white psychology's methodology and conclusions; and providing Afrocentric models for study, theory and therapy'.

Black psychology is as complex and diverse as the people it attempts to describe and understand. A wide range of models, theories, and approaches is used to describe the black psychological experience.

Karenga (1982) identified three schools of black psychology: the traditional school, the reformist school, and the radical school. The traditional school (for example, the work of Clark, 1965; Grier and Cobbs, 1968) is defined by: '(1) its defensive and/or reactive posture; (2) its lack of concern for the development of a Black psychology and its continued support for the Eurocentric model with minor changes; (3) its concern with changing white attitudes, and (4) its being essentially critical without substantial correctives' (Karenga, 1982: 325).

Among the significant contributors to the traditional school of black psychology are Grier, Cobbs, and Poussaint. In *Black Rage*, Grier and Cobbs (1968) argued that black people felt 'enraged' or experienced a sense of psychological rage as a consequence of inhumane and racist treatment. Nobles is critical of this work, and argues that Grier and Cobbs 'accepted uncritically the psychological principles available in western psychology as applicable to all people no matter what their race or cultural background' (Nobles, 1986: 70).

The reformist school (for example, White, 1980) is concerned about white attitudes and behaviours, 'but focuses more on change in public policy than on simply attitudinal change,' and, furthermore, 'begins to advocate an Afro-centric psychology, but combined with a traditional focus on change that would, ostensibly, benefit both blacks and whites ... (Thomas, 1971; Cross, 1971)' (Karenga, 1982: 325).

The radical school directs its attention 'to Black people in terms of analysis, treatment and transformation'. They 'insist on and are developing a psychology that has its roots in the African worldview (Jackson, 1982; King *et al.*, 1976)' (Karenga, 1982: 325).

There exists a tendency among black psychologists towards disagreement over whether the terms black and African have the same meaning, hence the concepts black psychology and African psychology. Some black psychologists suggest a basic distinction between the two concepts (Mosby, 1972; White, 1970, 1972; Williams, 1978), while others seem to use both concepts more or less synonymously (Akbar, 1975; Baldwin, 1976; Nobles, 1976). Some black psychologists who use the term black psychology rather exclusively also confine their focus to the African-American population. Others who use the term black psychology apply it to African (black) people generally (including African Americans). Jackson (1979) proposes that African psychology represents, more or less, the 'innovative-inventive' component of black psychology, which suggests that the former is subsumed under the latter (i.e., African psychology as a component of black psychology). From his survey of the definitional controversy among black psychologists, Jackson observed that:

> The appellate 'black psychology' is basically a generic designation for an emerging perspective in the field of psychology. Its embryonic stage of development is clearly illustrated in its range of definitions. At one extreme, Black psychology has been pictured not so much as a distinct academic discipline but as a reaction to an interpretation of psychology as a 'white' or Euro-centric endeavor .... At the other end of the continuum, some have hailed black psychology as the 'third great psychological-philosophical tradition with characteristic strengths and weaknesses ....' Much more reflective of the contemporary application of black psychology, Sims (1977) stated that it is 'concerned with redefining existing psychological principles and concepts, and developing additional models that will reveal the strengths of black people ... [it will] offer behavioral guidelines that have been examined in terms of their applicability to the specific needs and problems of black people' .... At the present time, it will be seen black psychology is a composite of reactive, inventive and innovative components and extends ... 'to the total behavior in all situations of black people throughout the world'.
>
> (Jackson, 1979: 271)

It is clear from this observation that black psychology is a combination of three components: reactive, inventive, and innovative, and deals with 'the total behaviour in all situations of black people throughout the world' (Jackson, 1979: 271).

I have already indicated that a wide range of models was used to describe black behaviour. Some of the models used were classified as follows: Africanity model, colonized/colonizer model, culture of poverty model, integritivistic model, and racial oppression model (Davis, 1982). These categories are not meant to be exclusive but were employed to facilitate a clearer understanding of the discipline of black psychology.

The Africanity model

This approach argues that African philosophy is potentially useful in helping us understand the behaviour of African Americans. The Africanity model attempts to explain black behaviour according to the tenets, values, and belief systems that derive from an African philosophical tradition. Several black scholars have argued that an African philosophical tradition should be the foundation of black psychology (Akbar, 1981, 2004; Nobles, 1972, 2004). They argue that recognition of the African roots of American blacks will produce a uniquely different understanding of black lifestyles and reality.

According to Nobles, 'African (Black) Psychology is rooted in the nature of black culture which is based on particular indigenous (originally indigenous to African) philosophical assumptions' (Nobles, 1980: 31). He states that one's cultural worldview influences how one perceives reality. The African worldview espouses groupness, sameness, commonality, co-operation and collective responsibility. In contrast, the Euro-American worldview espouses individuality, uniqueness, difference, competition, separateness, and independence. Nobles maintains that:

> Black psychology must concern itself with the mechanism by which our African definition has been maintained and what value its maintenance has offered black people. Hence, the task of Black psychology is to offer an understanding of the behavioral definition of African philosophy and to document what, if any, modifications it has undergone during particular experiential periods.
>
> (Nobles, 1980: 35)

African psychology maintains that the essence of the human being is spiritual. The assumption in black psychology is that the best way to know what we know is through affect or feeling. Joseph White describes the culture of African Americans as a feeling-oriented culture. White says 'In a feeling-oriented culture, apparent and when examined closely, superficial, logical contradictions do not have the same meaning as they might have in the Anglo culture' (White, 1972: 46).

An article entitled 'Vodoo or IQ: an introduction to African psychology' is considered to be an important work in the field of African psychology. The authors claim that 'one of the distinguishing characteristics of African as opposed to Euro-American psychology is the (utilitarian) end which is sought. The end of African psychology is the improvement of Africans (blacks), whereas the end of Euro-American psychology is to improve the lives of Euro-Americans (whites)' (Khatib et al., 1975: 13). The authors cite the differences between white and black people in the assumptions white people hold about themselves and the world. Some of the assumptions listed are:

1   that the world is basically material as opposed to spiritual;
2   that the black man is basically inferior to the white man;

3   that the 'self' is independent of other 'selves' and the environment;
4   that black people and white people can be measured by the same
    yardstick in terms of behaviour.

(Khatib *et al.*, 1979: 66–7)

Colonized/colonizer model

The colonized/colonizer model suggests that black (American) behaviour can be explained in terms of black people's history as a colonized people. This model proposes that blacks do not have unique behavioural patterns, but have similar patterns to other colonized people in the world. For example, Blauner (1969) argues that, although there are variations in the political and social structure of European colonialism and American slavery, they both developed out of a similar balance of technological, cultural, and power relations, and thus a common process of social oppression characterized the racial patterns in the contexts.

Culture of poverty model

The culture of poverty (or social class) model posits that the black 'predicament' is primarily a function of low socio-economic statuses, and that blacks in the lower economic state exhibit behavioural patterns similar to other lower social class groups.

Cultural integritivistic model

The cultural integritivistic model (Boykin, 1981) asserts that the cultural strengths and integrity of blacks should be expounded upon, and should be the conceptual framework for research in black psychology. Cross's (1971) model of psychological nigrescence is an example of this model. This model will be discussed in Chapter 5.

The racial oppression model

According to the racial oppression model, most of black behaviour is a response to living in a racist and oppressive society and has evolved out of the slavery experience. An example of this model can be seen in the work of Grier and Cobbs (1968). They argue that black Americans are filled with 'Black rage' after years of trying to survive in a racist, oppressive society. In order to survive, blacks have had to develop 'cultural paranoia', where every white person is considered to be an enemy until proven otherwise.

We can see that a number of different models have been used to explain black behaviour. For example, the colonizer and culture of poverty models do not view black behaviour as unique when compared with groups who find themselves in similar states of oppression, and, as such, do not consider black culture an important variable in their conceptualization of black life. However, some of the other models – the Africanity and integritivistic models, and to a lesser extent the racial oppression model – would consider black culture the cornerstone of black psychological research.

More recently, Jones (2004) notes that there has not been sufficient work by African American scholars across the various fields to develop a completely workable black psychology – a task that is ongoing. Four themes that have relevance for understanding contemporary black behaviour are: African philosophy; the African worldview; spirituality and religion; and the concept of resilience (Nobles, 2004; Jones, 2004). These themes 'do not exclusively undergrid all of African American/African/black life, but it does appear that they are important components of such behaviour ….our challenge is to establish the validity of these four constructs ... for understanding Black behaviour' (Jones, 2004: 55).

Differences between Western and black psychology

In the last three decades 'Black psychology has moved from invisibility to visibility' (White, 2004: 13). There have been 'major theoretical developments, research and research applications, extensions into ethnic psychology, and a call for cross-cultural competencies in the training and continuing education of psychologists' (White, 2004: 13). This section aims to describe briefly some differences between Western and black psychology in the study of the self and motivation.

The Eurocentric and black psychological approaches differ in terms of how they define the self. Western psychology is concerned with the study of the individual ego, behaviour, and consciousness. Thus, from a Freudian (psychoanalytic approach) to a Skinnerian (behaviourist) psychology, there is a common emphasis on individual differences as being the best description of human experience.

In contrast, black psychology describes this area of study as being the collective experience of oppression. Consequently, what must be studied to understand the human experience is the shared experience of oppression. The degree to which one is conscious of shared oppression is assumed to be a measure of 'black awareness' or 'black personality'. Therefore, we get models of black personality such as the Cross

(1971, 1995) model which describes development of black personality as growing from 'Negro to Black' conversion (see Chapter 5).

This approach, which begins to see personality as a collective phenomenon, is a critical contribution of black psychology. It makes a radical departure from the European-American preoccupation with the individual and his/her isolated experience. This is highlighted by Holdstock (2001). He notes that:

> An aspect of the revisioning of ourselves will have to be consideration of the competitive individualism that has thus far been the hallmark of contemporary psychology. We cannot expect a new world order to come about if we continue to endorse a concept of the self as a closed and self-sufficient unit of the social system. If we, as a select group of professionals who specialise in human behaviour, mental health, [and the actualization of the potential of individuals] fail to endorse an alternative, interdependent concept of the self that is more facilitative of achieving the ideals we aspire towards, then we have little hope of bringing about any change in society.
>
> (Holdstock, 2001: 204)

Another area of difference in the approaches of Western and black psychology is in the study of human motivation. The Eurocentric approach sees the person as essentially directed towards pleasurable gratification. The behaviourists assume that all behaviour hinges on rewards and punishments. Freud assumes the primal need of immediate gratification of either sexual or aggressive drives and Maslow assumes a hierarchy of needs for gratification at various levels. All these schools converge in the shared assumption that the critical goal of human personality is the desire for gratification.

The emphasis of black psychology is that the essential goal of human behaviour is survival. Various authors have emphasized the survival skills of black people as being the primary goal and accomplishment of personality (for example, White, 1991, 2004). The constant confrontation with racism and oppression is viewed as the consistent reality, and the development of strategies to outmanoeuvre threats to survival by black people is the goal of personality. Staples (1974) builds his theory of the black family on a survival-adaptation basis. His assumption is that confrontation with slavery and subsequent oppression shaped the African-American family through its struggles to survive.

Eurocentric standards of what constitutes mental health are often inappropriate for blacks because they are based on the philosophies, values, and mores of Euro-American culture, and these variables are used to develop normative standards of mental health. Akbar (1981) developed a new criterion for optimal mental functioning or 'normality' in black populations. He defined mental health as the 'affirmative identification and commitment of one's African (natural) identity'. He proposed a classification system of mental disorders (i.e., alien self-disorder; anti-self disorder; self-destructive disorder; and organic disorder) which demonstrate disordered behaviour to be a result of getting involved in behaviours which deny one's African identity. Akbar's classification system assumes that mental disorders and unnatural human behaviour are the results of inhuman conditions associated with racist oppression. His classification system is discussed in Chapter 7.

Cross-cultural psychology

In recent years, black psychology has become part of ethnic or cross-cultural psychology (Jones, 2004). In the USA, Asian American and Hispanic psychologists have developed ethnically oriented theories, research strategies and practical applications. The move toward 'ethnic [or cross-cultural] psychology has generated a demand for all psychologists to develop cross-cultural competencies, especially those who teach or work directly with ethnically diverse clients' (Jones, 2004: 14).

A number of psychologists in the USA called for the inclusion of cross-cultural approaches to Western psychology (e.g. Segall, Lonner and Berry, 1998; Matsumoto, 2001). However, in Britain there is a lack of research from a cross-cultural perspective. Segall, Dasen, Berry and Poortinga (1990) define cross-cultural psychology as 'the scientific study of human behaviour and its transmission, taking into account the ways in which the behaviors are shaped and influenced by social and cultural forces' (1990: 1). The study of ethnic groups and minorities within culturally plural societies is just as much a part of cross-cultural psychology as the study of widely varying and geographically dispersed cultural groups.

Black psychology has also addressed the question of culture (see Akbar, 1984; Baldwin, 1984; Boykin, 1994). Various authors (e.g. Boykin, 1994, 1997; Nsamenang, 1995; Shade, 1991) have examined the effects of African and African American culture on the development of black children. For example, Nsamenang's (1995) research explores the effects of differing cultural contexts on the socialization of African children and Shade's (1991) research on African American social cognition argues empirically that cognitive style, in which people organize and understand their world, is culturally induced, further arguing that African Americans have a distinctive cognitive style that should be embraced, understood, and appreciated.

Berry, *et al.* (1992) proposed three goals for the field of cross-cultural psychology: the first goal involves testing or extending the generalizability of existing theories and findings. Berry and Dasen (1974) referred to this as the 'transport and test goal' in which hypotheses and findings from one culture are transported to another so that their validity can be tested in other cultural settings or groups. For example, are the stages of cognitive development proposed by Jean Piaget specific to certain types of cultures, or are they universal? The second goal focuses on exploring other cultures in order to discover variations in behaviour that may not be part of one's own cultural experience. In other words, if findings cannot be generalized, what are the reasons for this, and are there behaviours unique to these other cultures? The third goal – which follows from the first two – is aimed at integrating findings in such a way as to generate a more universal psychology applicable to a wider range of cultural settings and societies.

Jahoda and Dasen (1986: 413), in their introduction to the special issue of the *International Journal of Behavioural Development*, called for a 'Cross-cultural developmental psychology .... [which] is not just comparative [but] essentially is an outlook that takes culture seriously' and deplored the fact that 'theories and findings in developmental psychology originating in the First world tend to be disseminated to the Third World as gospel truth'.

How can a cross-cultural perspective contribute to our understanding of human development? Gardiner (2004) has pointed to a number of important benefits. First, looking at behaviour from this perspective compels researchers to seriously reflect on the variety of ways in which their cultural beliefs and values affect the development of their theories and research designs. Second, increased awareness of cross-cultural findings provides an opportunity to extend or restrict the implications of research conducted in a single cultural group, most notably the United States and similar Western societies. Third, reduced ethnocentrism – by looking at behaviours as it occurs in another culture. It is important to note that the study of ethnic groups and minorities within culturally plural societies is just as much a part of cross-cultural psychology as the study of widely varying and geographically dispersed cultural groups.

One way of conceptualizing principles in cross-cultural studies is by using the analytical concepts of emics, etics, and theorics (Berry, 1969). Etics refer to aspects of life that appear to be consistent across different cultures; that is, etics refer to universal or pancultural truths or principles. Emics, in contrast, refer to aspects of life that appear to be different across cultures; emics, therefore, refer to truths or principles that are culture-specific (Berry, 1969). Etics that are assumed, but have not been demonstrated, to be true universals have been called imposed etics (Berry, 1969: 124). Such etics are said to be usually only Euro-American emics indiscriminately, even ethnocentrically, imposed on the interpretation of behaviour in other cultures. A true etic, in contrast, is empirically and theoretically derived from the common features of a phenomenon under investigation in different cultures. Berry (1969: 124) called this a derived etic. Berry (1980: 13) defined theorics as 'theoretical concepts employed by social scientists to interpret and account for emic variation and etic constancies'. A cross-cultural psychology that relies solely or primarily on Euro-American concepts cannot be expected to achieve its stated aims. However, 'there is a paucity of theorizing with the use of concepts that are non-Western origin' (1980: 9).

Etic versus emic goals provides social workers with a theoretical framework for working with culturally diverse children and young people and adults. Poortinga (1997: 352) states: 'Behavior is emic or culture specific, to the extent it can only be understood within the cultural context within which it occurs; it is etic, or universal, in as much as it is common to human beings independent of their culture'. It follows that when a researcher or observer assumes that his or her own emic-etic distinction is true for all cultures, she/he is operating from an ethnocentric point of view and that cultural misunderstanding will result. For example, in the case of Erikson's theory, the development of autonomy and independence (the emic) "fits" well with Western cultural values.

Implications for social work practice

Research knowledge and information from a black psychological perspective on black family life, black mental health, and black lifestyles are vital to the social work profession. However, in Britain there is a lack of research from a black perspective. Ahmad points out that 'the current marginalization of the black perspective can only be overcome if white society is able and willing to challenge orthodox research assumptions' (Ahmad, 1989: 155).

We need to develop instruments to measure black behaviour in Britain. We rely on measures that were developed for and standardized on white populations. We must question whether it is always appropriate to use such measures to study black behaviour and experience.

A Eurocentric perspective in psychology has meant certain theoretical deficits when social workers attempt to apply it in practice. Traditional psychology perpetuates a notion of deviance with respect to black people. Social workers may be prone to making certain assumptions in their assessments on the basis of these stereotypes. An alternative to focusing on stereotypes or pathological characteristics of black groups is to emphasize the black client's cultural assets and strengths, such as the abilities to cope with stress, to implement survival skills, and to use extended family and community support systems. There is a need for social workers (and social work students) to identify the strengths of black families and utilize these strengths in their work with black clients (Graham, 2007).

Weaver declares:

> Search for strengths relates to the social worker's emphasis on positive aspects of individual and family systems. It is crucial to begin with strengths of the family system: families move on strengths, not weaknesses. There are inherent strengths in the design of every family; the social worker must help the family use their own strengths in making choices and decisions that will enable them to achieve their desired goal. This skill, as it relates to the search for and use of strength within the family system, has the potential for being very empowering.
>
> (Weaver, 1982: 103)

An understanding of the black perspective in psychology helps social workers to assess the problems of black clients more accurately and to develop solutions and appropriate intervention techniques. There is a need for social workers to study what is 'effective for black people', that is, studying black people who have coped effectively and building norms for behaviour based on that coping rather than comparing it with white norms. Sue (2006) encourages a focus on strengths, resources, and potential in the client and his or her environment rather than on problem pathology. The ethnically sensitive social worker starts with the assumption that many minority problems are rooted in a racist society.

An understanding of cross-cultural psychology can help social workers towards developing culturally competent practice. According to Sue and Sue (1999: 110) 'To become a culturally skilled helper [practitioner], one must ... acquire knowledge of culturally diverse groups that will pave the way for grasping the worldviews of culturally different clients, and develop a range of intervention strategies and skills that are appropriate, relevant, and sensitive to diverse groups'.

Conclusion

Black psychology emerged from the kinds of negative statements about black people which have characterized the vast majority of the European-American psychological literature. Psychological practices in Britain and the United States have been white dominated and are often culturally biased and racist. Although white psychologists claimed that they were objective scientists, they defined black people from a point of view that focused on defectiveness and pathology. A black psychological perspective challenges the Eurocentric theoretical formulations and research paradigms that have a potentially oppressive effect on black people. It attempts to build a theoretical model that organizes, explains, and leads to understanding the behaviour of black people.

However, developments in black and cross-cultural perspectives in psychology are more advanced in the USA than in Britain. To the extent that the goal of a black perspective in psychology is to try to understand the behaviour of black people, there is a need in Britain for black psychologists and researchers to concentrate on developing paradigms and models that will more accurately depict the reality of black psychological experience.

2 Forming impressions of people
A black perspective

Introduction

Rosaldo reports: 'Cities throughout the world today increasingly include minorities defined by race, ethnicity, language, class, religion, and sexual orientation. Encounters with "difference" now pervade modern everyday life in urban settings' (Rosaldo, 1989: 28). This chapter examines, some of the factors involved in impression formation from a black perspective. Psychology texts for social workers (for example, Nicolson, Bayne and Owen, 2006) fail to address the black perspective in impression formation. A good example to consider is cultural differences in eye-contact behaviour. Interactions between members of different cultures may be problematic if the meaning of the behaviour is misinterpreted (Argyle, 1988; Matsumoto, 2001). Other differences between cultures include factors such as people's use of personal space (for example, how close it is appropriate to stand in conversation with another person); touch (for example, when and how often you touch another person), eye-contact behaviour and perception of time (Argyle, 1990; Matsumoto, 2001). This chapter also explores differences in communication styles between high and low context cultures (Hall, 1976).

As discussed in Chapter 1, general psychology has failed to provide a full and accurate understanding of the black reality. Most of the research is Eurocentric in theory, method, and focus. Eurocentric theories are derived from European-American theories, conducted by whites about whites, and the results are assumed to be culture-general rather than culture-specific findings. For instance, the majority of systematic research on nonverbal behaviour has used white middle-class college students as subjects. Fairchild and Edwards-Evans (1990) argue that: 'Because of the omnipresence of White racism (see Bowser & Hunt, 1981), much of the social sciences, including education, linguistics, and psychology, has revealed clear White racial biases concerning studies of African Americans [and other black groups] (see Fairchild & Gurin, 1978)' (Fairchild and Edward-Evans, 1990: 76).

In this chapter I argue that we need to examine impression formation from a black perspective, as white social workers working with black people may make judgements about them unaware that the behaviour they are observing has a cultural bias that they are misinterpreting.

In the following sections I will discuss some of the factors, identified in the psychological literature, which influence our impressions of people – from a black perspective. According to Ickes there are relatively 'few studies in the literature [on black-white relations] in which the actual social interactions of whites and blacks are examined' (Ickes, 1984: 330). Most of the existing research and literature in this area is US based. However, many of the findings are relevant to other non-white racial groups.

Perception

There probably is no subject matter more central to psychology than perception. Fellows has defined perception as 'the process by means of which an organism receives and analyses information' (Fellows, 1968: 218). Chaplin has defined perception as 'a group of sensations to which meaning is added from past experience' (Chaplin, 1975: 376). Samovar and Porter (2001: 14) have defined perception as 'the internal process by which we select, evaluate, and organize stimuli from the external environment'. These definitions describe two events in which we participate when interacting with our environment. First, we 'receive' information. This reception refers to sensation, or the process by which information comes to us through our senses. However, we do more than just receive or sense stimuli – we also analyse what we sense. Such an analysis process has two components – attention and organization (Fellows, 1968: 5). Attention refers to the process whereby we systematically choose those stimuli to which we will attend, as we cannot possibly sense all there is to be received in the environment. In order to make sense of the various elements we have selected, we must engage in a process of organization. Thus, we convert the experience of our sense receptors into a 'useful and consistent' (Fellows, 1968: 5) picture. Perception is an active not a passive process. It is one in which the perceiver adds his/her own meaning to the data provided by his/her senses (Samovar and Porter, 2005).

First impressions

As soon as we observe anything about a person, we begin to form an impression of that person. Of the many stimuli, we select only the more noticeable ones upon which to build our first impressions. Once we have formed this first impression, later observations will be influenced by our first impression. The first impression of a person determines our behaviour towards him/her. That person, in turn, behaves in a manner consistent with our behaviour, and this consequently reinforces our initial impression. For example, if a white social worker perceives a black client as hostile and responds to his/her own perception with defensiveness or hostility, the black client will tend to respond to the white social worker's response with hostility. Thus, the first impression of the white social worker is then confirmed, perhaps a self-fulfilled prophecy. The black client may have been hostile or friendly from the outset. However, the white social worker's predisposition to select any feature that could be interpreted as hostility, almost predestines the black client to grow into the hostile expectation of the white. First impressions are very difficult to change, even in the face of contradictory evidence. Nicolson, Bayne and Owen (2006) suggest that 'the most direct way of countering the disproportionate power of first impressions is first to become aware of them and then to treat them as hypotheses – to check the evidence on which they are based, and to look for further evidence' (2006: 95).

Stereotypes

The term 'stereotype' has been extensively used by laymen and academics from a wide variety of disciplines. Many of the viewpoints generally expressed in present-day literature regarding stereotypes originate as far back as 1922 with Walter Lippman, one of the first to define and employ the construct of the stereotype. Present-day literature has maintained Lippman's 'point that the "real environment" is too complex for us to understand it fully and directly, therefore we perceive the world more simply: stereotypes are part of this process of simplifying the world in order to be able to deal with it' (Hinton, 2000: 66). The process of stereotyping involves three stages:

> The first is identifying a set of people as a specific category ... [this might be] ... skin colour, sex, age .... The second stage involves assigning a range of characteristics to that category of people .... The final stage is the attribution of these characteristics to every

member of the category ... this overgeneralization ... brings out the prejudiced nature of stereotyping as all group members are placed in the 'strait jacket' of the stereotype.

(Hinton, 2000: 66)

The dynamics of stereotyping ascribe to a single individual the characteristics associated with a group of people, or extend to a group the characteristics attributed to a single individual. The stereotype generally represents a negative judgement of both the group and the individual, and emphasizes negative differences. For black people, negative stereotyping has revolved around skin colour, low intelligence, pathological behaviour, etc. Stereotyping occurs in the context of racism as a means of explaining away black people as inferior.

Findings on 'ethnic stereotyping show that in American [and British] society more negative characteristics are ascribed to persons of black and brown skin than persons with light or white skin colour' (Andrews and Majors, 2004: 319).

Social workers must note that the tendency to rely on stereotypes to ease the difficulty of interacting with the unfamiliar is very strong for all people, regardless of racial or ethnic identity. It is easier for us to draw on preconceptions when in doubt than it is to make the effort to seek out and know individuals. Although stereotypes are helpful in ordering the complexity of human experience (Hinton, 2000; Lippman, 1922; Matsumoto, 2001), they interfere with meaningful interaction, because they predispose to interaction between preconceptions rather than between the participants themselves.

Social workers need to be aware that, to any interracial communication situation, they will bring the capacity and predisposition to 'perceive' based on a combination of what really exists 'out there', and the set of expectations existing in 'the world inside our heads'. Social workers' prejudice will precondition them to respond to black clients in specific ways. Racial prejudice tends to define and circumscribe the interracial communication process. Stereotypic statements tend to ignore individual differences between ethnic group members and emphasize generalized and/or exaggerated traits of the group.

Paralanguage

Paralanguage deals with how something is said and not what is said. It deals with the range of nonverbal cues surrounding common speech behaviour (Knapp, 1978, 2006). Paralanguage includes all that accompanies language: pitch, range, rhythm, tempo and articulation;

vocalizations – vocal characterizers: laughing, crying, sighing, etc.; vocal qualifiers – intensity, pitch heights, extent. Other vocal cues include pauses, silences, dialect or accent, speech rate, duration of utterance and interaction rates. Paralanguage is very likely to be revealed in conversation conventions, such as how we greet, address and take turns in speaking.

Sue (2006: 162) notes that 'directness of conversation or the degree of frankness (paralanguage) varies among various cultural groups'. For instance, many Asians 'converse in an indirect or circular pattern, contrasting markedly with the direct, linear orientation of English [people]' (McAvoy and Sayeed, 1990: 61).

The most relevant element in paralanguage in terms of impression formation is the impact that accent or dialect patterns have upon social workers in the interview situation. Accents and dialects carry with them stereotypes of the speakers employing them, and these stereotypes affect the impressions social workers' form in interracial interaction. Many black people are not only physically stereotyped, but vocally stereotyped as well.

Clothing

Social workers need to be aware that black people's dress patterns, and the stereotypes associated with them, have an important impact on impression formation. While clothing may provide us with some information about a person, it also tends to block input of other information, by causing us to perceive selectively based on our stereotype of clothing patterns and personality types. In order to overcome this effect, social workers must engage in a dedicated effort consciously to fight the impact of these preconceptions about clothing.

Physical characteristics

Social workers not only stereotype on the basis of what others wear in terms of clothing, but also form stereotypes based on the actual physical characteristics of their clients. Culture dictates certain standards of beauty and those physical traits considered desirable; thus members of a culture respond to the physical make-up of each other in the pattern determined by the society. Thus, 'Whether warranted or not, the existence of such physical stereotypes will necessarily affect interpersonal perceptions' (Barnlund, 1968: 520).

Language

Black groups define themselves in part through language, and members establish identity through language use (White *et al.*, 2008). Black English is a distinctive language code. A Creole language or dialect, referred to as black English, has been identified as a distinctive language characteristic of black (African-American and African-Caribbean) culture (King and James, 1983; Labov, 1982). Black (African-Caribbean) people often feel the need to switch between their own cultural language code and that of the more dominant white society. There is a tendency among some authors to describe black English as a deviant or deficient form of mainstream or standard English (Smitherman, 1977, 2004; Smitherman-Donaldson, 1988). Viewing black English as a dialect stems from a Eurocentric perspective that describes only what is 'missing' and what is grammatically 'incorrect'. Therefore, we need to use the term black English, rather than black dialect, to indicate the language form. Black English is now recognized as a legitimate language form with a unique and logical syntax, semantic system and grammar (Jenkins, 1982; Smitherman, 1977, 2004; Smitherman-Donaldson, 1988) that varies in its forms depending upon which African language influenced it, and in which region it was developed (Smitherman, 1977). There is strong evidence of the African influence in both the early and current forms of black English (Smitherman, 1977, 2004, see Baugh, 1983, for detailed discussion). Speech that marks the individual as a member of the group can be important for in-group acceptance. Here the use of black language promotes identity and may be reinforced by group members. For African Americans black English represents group solidarity (Smitherman, 2004).

> Black English of the African American underclass is not only diverging from the White English, but from the English of the African American middle class as well. The children of the Black underclass are rejecting the bourgeois socio-linguistic character of the schools and dropping out or being forced out of school. At the same time the African American middle class is being jolted out of its complacency by the reemergence of racism.
>
> (Smitherman, 2004: 306)

Linguistic distinctiveness strategies are used by people when they identify strongly with their own group and are insecure about other groups (Giles and Johnson, 1981). In Britain Creole is used to establish in-group identity (Hewitt, 1986). For example, among some groups arguments produce increased use of Jamaican pronunciations. Teenagers seem to equate strength and assertiveness with Creole and use it strategically with authority figures such as police and social workers. Where there is a power differential, Creole use takes on political and cultural significance because it denotes assertiveness and group identity (Hewitt, 1986).

Racist attitudes to any language spoken by African Caribbean people, as well as the racist overtones and nuances of the English language itself, have contributed to the adoption of Creole by many second generation young African Caribbean people (Wong, 1986). For many African Caribbean adolescents, 'Patois is a powerful social and political mantle which ... becomes an aggressive and proud assertion of "racial" and class identities' (Wong, 1986: 119). Thus, the acquisition of competence in Creole is an expression of racial identity and solidarity as well as a demonstration of determination to acquire status and power (Wong, 1986). In a comparative study of two generations of African Caribbeans and Asians, Modood *et al.* (1994) explored the attitudes of first generation African Caribbeans toward the use and transmission of Creole and Patois languages. Half of the first generation of African Caribbeans in the sample felt that it was not important for them or their children to maintain an oral Creole or Patois tradition. Whereas, most of the second generation respondents in Modood *et al.*'s study felt that it was essential for African Caribbeans to be able to communicate in Creole and patois. They felt that it was important to maintain their oral tradition as part of their cultural identity. In choosing to focus on Creole, 'young black adolescents are refusing to be "standardised" and are refusing to be swallowed up by the more dominant white middle class culture' (Graham, 2000: 46).

Because of the stigma attached by the dominant culture to nonstandard dialects and forms, it is difficult for black people to use black English. The dominant white culture has selected mainstream white English as preferred usage and relegated other forms – black English – to nonstandard, lower-prestige status (Jenkins, 1982; Seymour and Seymour, 1979). Social workers need to be aware that the dominant white society's rejection of black English as a legitimate linguistic style may influence their perceptions of clients speaking black English.

Nonverbal communication

Nonverbal communication 'is the likely basis of many first impressions' (Nicolson, Bayne and Owen, 2006: 100). In a classic study Mehrabian and Ferris (1967) demonstrated that nonverbal behaviour is an important source of information. The authors indicated that impressions were formed more strongly through (nonverbal) speech (38 per cent) and facial features (55 per cent), than through verbal content (7 per cent). We tend to regard nonverbal communication as the 'true' indicator of a communicator's meaning, because nonverbal behaviour (frequently unconscious or reflexive) is more difficult to control than verbal behaviour. Therefore, our true emotions will often 'leak' through in hints of nervousness, anger, boredom and other feelings. If white practitioners 'are unaware of their own biases, the nonverbals are most likely to reveal their true feelings' (Sue and Sue, 2003: 62). In order to survive in a white-dominated society, black people have 'to rely on nonverbal cues more often than verbal ones' (2003: 62). Thus, if white social workers have not dealt adequately with their own racism, the black client will be quick to detect any racist biases.

Research into nonverbal behaviour is of two types, related either to studying the meaning attributed to nonverbal behaviour or to assessing its frequency (Gudykunst, 2004). However, the research on nonverbal behaviour and communication in black culture has been limited. The purpose of this section is to discuss the significance of nonverbal behaviours and communication among black people. We need to be aware that:

> Cultural differences in nonverbal behaviour can ... be a source of miscommunication (LaFrance and Mayo, 1978). Also, if someone does not behave in an expected manner then ... the perceiver might be tempted to make an internal attribution. [Hence] in a society where there is limited emotional expression a member of a more expressive culture might be inferred to be 'over-emotional'.
>
> (Hinton, 2000: 155)

Two influential articles on black American nonverbal behaviours and communication are 'Black kinesics: some nonverbal communication patterns in Black culture' (Johnson, 1971) and 'Nonverbal communication among Afro-Americans: an initial classification' (Cooke, 1980, originally published in 1972). These articles were written during the predominance of the black power movement. In the US, 'the black power movement, reflected "a period of symbolism", i.e., a period when Black Americans more often than not used nonverbal behaviours and communication styles in clothes, handshakes, hairstyles, stance, walking styles, etc., to symbolize power, struggle, anger, strength, protest, defiance, unity, pride, independence, and solidarity' (Andrews and Majors, 2004: 273) (see Cooke, 1980). However, 'many nonverbal behaviours in African American culture have changed to reflect today's needs, taken on new forms, or have disappeared altogether' (Andrews and Majors, 2004: 273).

White (1984, 1999), in emphasizing the rich oral tradition of Africans and African Americans, recounted in some detail the verbal and nonverbal rituals found in many African-American communities. Others have noted the importance of nonverbal cues in conveying or modifying the meaning of the spoken word (Baugh, 1983; Cooke, 1980).

The majority of researchers in the field of nonverbal communication categorize nonverbal communication into the following areas: kinesics or body movements (i.e. gestures, movements of the body, e.g. hands, limbs, head, feet, and legs); facial expressions (smiles); eye behaviour (blinking, direction and length of gaze, and pupil dilation); posture, touching behaviour (stroking, hitting, holding); paralanguage (vocal qualities, e.g. pitch, tempo, etc.) and nonlanguage sounds (moans, yells, etc.); physical characteristics (physique, body shape, general attractiveness, body or breath odours, hair, weight, height, and skin colour); proxemics (people's use and perception of personal and social space); artefacts (perfume, clothes, spectacles, etc.); and environmental factors (architecture, furniture, lighting, crowding, music and noise, smells, weather, or related factors that could affect the communication process).

Before discussing some of the above dimensions of nonverbal communication, I wish to focus briefly on the impact of racism and discrimination on black people's presentation of self to others and impression management. We must not underestimate the impact of discrimination and racism on the 'way in which Black people relate to each other and to the outside world .... Skin color ... is a badge of difference. The process of discrimination is evident at all levels of society [with] theories about genetic inferiority (Jensen, 1969) and cultural pathology (Moynihan, 1965)' (Boyd-Franklin, 2003: 10). Few, if any, black individuals can live in Britain and the US and not be affected by racism and discrimination.

Black people often see nonverbal messages as more credible than verbal messages. When a contradiction occurs between the verbal and nonverbal messages, black people tend to believe the nonverbal messages more. A common saying among African Americans is: 'If you really want to know what White folks are thinking and feeling, don't listen to what they say, but how they say it'. Such a statement refers to the biases, stereotypes, and racist attitudes that whites are believed to possess, but that they consciously or unconsciously conceal' (Sue and Sue, 1999: 60). In discussing nonverbal communication among black people, Boyd-Franklin (2003: 178) used the term 'vibes' as follows: 'black people, because of the often extremely subtle ways in which racism manifests itself socially, are particularly attuned to very fine distinctions among such variables in all interactions ... Because of this, many [black people] have been socialized to pay attention to all of the nuances of behaviour and not just to the verbal message.

We need not only to understand how black people react to and express distrust towards white people but also to have an understanding of nonverbal behaviours (and communication styles) among blacks. As discussed in Chapter 7, black people's anger and distrust towards white people could be viewed as appropriate, adaptive behaviour (Grier and Cobbs, 1968). In the US, it appears that certain nonverbal behaviours in black Americans have taken on unique characteristics as a consequence of the 'history of conflict' with white people in the country (for example, slavery, racism, discrimination). For this reason, Andrews and Majors (2004) consider that 'survival, pride, solidarity, camaraderie, entertainment, and bitterness have become the impetus for and raison d'être of many culture-specific nonverbal behaviors in present day African American culture' (Andrews and Majors, 2004: 320). They also argue that, in order:

> To cope with the 'invisibility' and frustration resulting from racism and discrimination, many African American people have channeled their creative talents and energies into the construction and use of particular expressive and conspicuous styles of nonverbal behaviours (e.g., in their demeanour, gestures, clothing, hairstyles, walk, stances, and handshakes, among other areas). For many African American people these unique, expressive, colorful, stylish and performance-oriented behaviours are ways to act 'cool', to be visible and show pride. Elsewhere these behaviours have been referred to as 'Coolpose' (Collias, 1988, Doyle, 1989 ...).
>
> (Andrews and Majors, 2004: 316)

Messinger *et al.* (1962; as cited in Majors, 1991) provide us with a good example of how black people use different roles because of their distrust of white people and in an attempt to survive. They quote Sammy Davis, Jr. as saying, 'As soon as I go out the front door of my house in the morning, I'm on ... but when I'm with the group, I can relax. We trust each other.' Thus, 'there are times when, although "off stage", he [Davis] felt "on-stage".' The authors conclude with a citation from another author, Bernard Wolfe, who asserts that we can most probably expect 'members of any oppressed group [to have] similar experiences'

(Majors, 1991: 74). It is highly probable that black people in Britain have similar experiences. From this perspective, black people will regard presentations of self to others and impression management as the key to control and survival.

High and low context

Hall (1976) proposed the concept of high and low context cultures. In low context cultures (for example, the US and Britain), verbal messages are elaborate and highly specific, and tend also to be highly detailed and redundant. Verbal abilities are highly valued. Low context cultures have been associated with being more opportunistic, more individual rather than group oriented (Sue, 2006). In high context cultures, most of the information is either in the physical context, or internalized in the person. Very little is in the coded, explicit, and transmitted part of the message. High context cultures are more sensitive to nonverbal messages; hence they are more likely to provide a context and setting and let the point evolve. Black cultures have been described as high context. Many black people require fewer words than their white counterparts to communicate the same content (Sue, 2006). Asian Americans, African Americans, Hispanics and other minority groups in the US emphasize high context cues. Sue (2006: 164) observes that 'the fact that African Americans may communicate more by HC [high context] cues has led many to characterize them as nonverbal, inarticulate, unintelligent ...'.

This notion of context poses problems when social work clients are from cultures that differ in context level. When social workers (from low context cultures) interact with clients of high context cultures (African Asian), the social workers are liable to have difficulty in communicating because the high context messages do not contain sufficient information for practitioners to gain a true or complete meaning. Social workers may interpret a high context culture message according to their low context disposition, and reach entirely the wrong meaning. People in high context cultures have an expectation that others are also able to understand the unarticulated communication; hence, they do not speak as much as people from low context cultures. Thus, what is not said may be more important in determining meaning than what is said.

Low and high context communication exists in all cultures, but one tends to predominate (Hall, 1976). Understanding that a client is from a high or low context culture, and the form of communication that predominates in these cultures, will make the black client's behaviour less confusing and more interpretable to the practitioner.

Visual behaviour

A major nonverbal facial feature relates to maintaining eye contact in a dyad or to 'gaze behaviour': looking at or looking away from the person being addressed. This section is concerned with visual behaviour, which is one of the most studied aspects of nonverbal behaviour.

In African-American nonverbal behaviour, visual behaviour (eye contact, gaze, staring, etc.) plays a major role. In particular, it plays an important role in interpersonal communication, interpersonal attraction, and arousal. Andrews and Majors (2004) point out that recent research on visual behaviour among African Americans has been minimal.

The research carried out by LaFrance and Mayo (1976) demonstrates that black Americans tend to have lower eye contact and gaze than whites. These authors suggest that white authority figures (e.g., administrators, teachers, educators, etc.) often misread black American eye behaviour (for example, inferring that black people are uninterested, less honest, withhold information, and have poor concentration). According to LaFrance and Mayo, it is important to use a cultural framework when interpreting eye contact and gaze. White people tend to associate eye contact and eye gaze with affiliation, positive attitudes between communicators, trustworthiness, forthrightness, and sincerity (Hanna, 1984; Matsumoto, 2006). Black people, on the other hand, may associate eye contact and gaze with negative overtones and a lack of respect. Hanna's (1984) data also showed some black Americans were reluctant to look directly in the eye of persons who occupied an authority position.

Hemsley and Doob (1978) investigated the relation between credibility and gaze behaviour in an experimental setting. Subjects were exposed to film fragments depicting a witness in court. In one fragment the witness looked directly at the judge while testifying; in the other the witness gazed at the floor. The content of the testimonies was identical. Results showed that the testimony was perceived to be more credible if the witness maintained eye contact with the judge. These reviews generally reveal a consistent pattern of meanings attributed to gaze behaviour. Individuals who frequently look their discussion partner in the eye are not only considered to be more credible, but are also judged to be more congenial, attentive, competent, more skilful socially, and more assertive. In sum, frequent and sustained eye contact is systematically judged more positively than looking away. It should be noted that these studies all relate to white participants and subjects and are therefore 'white culture' oriented.

Research on eye contact across race generally shows that African Americans look at others while listening with less frequency than whites (Smith, 1983; Harper *et al.*, 1978; Hanna, 1984). White people tend to look at others more when listening than speaking, whereas black people do the opposite (Hanna, 1984). It has been found that black parents sometimes teach their children that looking an adult in the eye is a sign of disrespect (Byers and Byers, 1972). In contrast, white children are socialized to do just the opposite: looking away from a speaker is seen as disrespectful.

Overall, LaFrance and Mayo (1976) found that looking while listening occurred least for black males and most for white females. The eye and visual literature shows that, overall, females use eye contact more frequently than males (Smith, 1983).

Research into the meaning of gaze behaviour within the black culture is rare, so that definite conclusions cannot be made. However, Garratt *et al.* (1981) and Ickes (1984) provide some empirical evidence that the meaning attributed to gaze behaviour in the culture of blacks contrasts with the usual white attributions. Garratt *et al.* made an inventory of the style of police questioning preferred by black and white subjects. The results suggest that white subjects prefer a police officer to look at them during questioning, while blacks do not. Blacks experience frequent eye contact as impolite. Ickes moreover notes that blacks consider continued eye contact as provoking, arrogant, and disdainful. Black people may appear to be indifferent or uninvolved in their interactions with whites (Asante and Noor-Aldee, 1984; Ickes, 1984). European Americans are more likely to experience such interactions as somewhat difficult and burdensome and therefore tend to talk, look at the other, and smile more (Ickes, 1984). He concludes that, compared to blacks, European Americans either anticipate or perceive greater difficulty and awkwardness in these initial interracial interactions, and feel a particular responsibility and concern for making the interaction work. These patterns may reflect over-accommodation on the part of European Americans (Giles and Coupland, 1991).

Eye-contact patterns may account for some of the disparities in level of involvement in conversations between white social workers and black clients. Some European Americans interpret the nonverbal behaviour of a person who does not look at them at all in conversation as being inattentive (Kleinke, 1986; Matsumoto, 2006). On the other hand, the behaviour of a person who looks at them during conversation is interpreted as interested. European Americans may interpret the behaviour of a person from another culture as inattentive or rude due to the differences between cultures in gaze behaviour (Argyle, 1988;

Manusov and Patterson, 2006). When European Americans speak they tend to look at their partner less than they do while listening (Atkinson *et al.*, 1979; Kendon, 1967; LaFrance and Mayo, 1976). For blacks this pattern is reversed, with listeners looking less and speakers looking more (LaFrance and Mayo, 1976). Consequently, white people look less and blacks look more while speaking. But while listening, whites look more and blacks look less. When these patterns are combined we can anticipate that when a European American is speaking the individuals interacting (interactants) will not be looking at each other frequently. This may be interpreted as boredom, lack of interest, and low involvement by a social worker or other white professional interviewing black clients. When a black person is speaking, there is more mutual eye contact than either would expect (LaFrance and Mayo, 1976) and this may be interpreted as intensity, hostility, or power. Ickes (1984) suggests that 'A common outcome of this clash of cultural expectations is that black and white participants both experience their visual interaction as somewhat awkward and uncomfortable' (Ickes, 1984: 331).

Ethnic differences in gaze behaviour have been demonstrated almost exclusively in American research. These differences, then, apply particularly to American whites and non-whites. Does such ethnic variation also occur in Europe?

Winkel and Vrij (1990) studied the frequency and effects of gaze behaviour in cross-cultural interactions between police officers and civilians (Dutch and Surinamers) in the Netherlands. The first part of the study showed that Surinamers make less eye contact during questioning than Dutch subjects do. This finding is similar to US studies on ethnic differences in gaze behaviour. In addition, Surinamers' degree of integration into Dutch society did not affect their gaze behaviour, suggesting this behavioural pattern to be stable. The Dutch subjects assessed black gaze behaviour more negatively and evaluated citizens displaying black gaze behaviour as more suspect, less congenial, and more tense.

The nonverbal behaviour of Surinamers leaves police officers with a negative impression. The frequent complaint, cited by Aalberts and Kamminga (1983), among officers that 'they' (Surinamers) are always lying because 'they never look you in the eye' is a telling illustration of this. It is evident that 'it does not take much of a departure from the white norm to influence impression formation in a way that is disadvantageous to Surinamers' (Winkel and Vrij, 1990).

Winkel and Vrij's (1990) study indicates that white police officers do commit nonverbal communication errors. A white officer, questioning a black civilian, will find the latter averting his eyes a great deal. Although the black person may do this, say, to show respect, the white officer might erroneously interpret it as indicative of untrustworthiness or rudeness. Other studies (Rozelle and Baxter, 1975; Kraut and Poe, 1980) moreover showed that in forming impressions of other people, police officers rely heavily on nonverbal information.

Various reviews indicate that non-whites and whites differ not only in attributing meanings to gaze behaviour, but also in the performance of that behaviour. Research conducted in the United States shows that in conversations white partners look at one another more frequently than non-whites usually do (Smith, 1983; Ickes, 1984). These studies indicate that during a conversation whites look at their partners for 55 per cent of the time, compared with 42 per cent for blacks – which amounts to 33 seconds per minute for whites and 25 seconds per minute in the case of non-whites. Kadushin notes that Native Americans and American Asians also 'tend to regard eye contact as disrespectful; restraint in the use of eye contact is regarded as a sign of deference. There is a greater use of peripheral vision' (Kadushin, 1990: 288).

In Asian cultures, direct eye-to eye contact is avoided during a conversation, particularly if the other person is of the opposite sex; this behaviour should not be taken as avoidance of the issue being discussed. For example, among Muslim women 'sitting with somewhat bowed head and downcast eyes is a sign of great modesty' (McAvoy and Sayeed, 1994: 61). In Britain a person who fails to establish eye contact is often seen as being evasive or unassertive (Mercer, 1984).

One study showed that Arabs, Latin Americans and Southern Europeans focused their gaze on the eyes or face of their conversational partner, whereas Asians, Indians and Pakistanis tend to show peripheral gaze or no gaze at all (Harper *et al.*, 1978).

A further difference between blacks and whites relates to the use of 'back-channel' behaviours, which are the short sounds that listeners make during conversation to indicate that they are listening to what the speaker is saying. The typical back-channel pattern for white listeners is to nod their heads, accompanying the nods with verbal responses such as 'um-hum'. Black listeners, in contrast, use either head nodding or a verbal response to indicate that they are attending to what the speaker is saying (Erickson, 1976).

Differences in white and black visual behaviour have clear applications to the social work interview. Instead of assuming that the client's averted eyes indicate lack of understanding, a social worker more familiar with patterns of black nonverbal behaviour might well attribute it to a culturally learned behaviour pattern. Differences in nonverbal behaviour, both in terms of the kinds of behaviour carried out and how such behaviour is decoded, may occur between whites and blacks.

Touching

There are race and gender differences in touching behaviour (Smith, 1983). It appears that females use touching more for intimacy and friendship, while males use touching more for status and power (Eakins and Eakins, 1978; Smith, 1983).

People in collectivistic cultures (such as Asian, African and African Caribbean) tend to engage in more tactile interaction than people in individualistic cultures (see Robinson, 1998 for discussion of collectivistic and individualistic cultures). Black Americans touch other blacks more than they touch European Americans, and this is even more evident after successes in sports (Halberstadt, 1985; Smith *et al.*, 1980). Smith *et al.*, for example, found a higher rate of touching among Black Americans than whites in expression of congratulations on a bowling team. This pattern is particularly true of lower socioeconomic class black Americans. In a study of touching behaviour, Hall (1974) found that working-class blacks, as opposed to middle-class whites and working-class Hispanics, showed a greater tendency towards bodily contact in interpersonal interactions. It has also been observed that interracial dyads touch less than intraracial dyads among both European Americans and black Americans (Willis *et al.*, 1976). Interracial touching is less highly valued by black people (Blubaugh and Pennington, 1976).

Race research on touching behaviours has shown that black Americans, as contrasted with whites, touch others in a wider variety of different situations. Heinig (1975) reported that black American students touched teachers more than their white counterparts. Willis *et al.*, (1976) showed that touching behaviour among black Americans was much greater than the touching behaviour among white children (Hanna, 1984). In a study of touching behaviours among black Americans and white female pairs, Willis and Hoffman (1975) observed that there was 'more frequent touching in same sex and same race dyads than in dyads of other race/sex combinations' (Smith, 1983: 58). Willis *et al.*, (1976) found that touching was more likely to occur in black-black dyads with females touching more frequently than any other group. Black females use touching behaviours in order to communicate intimacy (Willis *et al.*, 1976). Class differences in touching have also been found, with people in higher-income groups touching less than those in lower-income groups (Henley, 1977).

Time

Chronemics is the study of how we perceive, structure, use and react to time. It includes perceptions of when someone is 'on time' and the significance of being 'late'. Our perception of time is culturally determined and differs greatly among different groups.

The study of meanings, usage and communication of time is probably the most discussed and well-researched nonverbal code in the intercultural literature (Hall, 1984; Gudykunst and Kim, 1997). According to Poyatos (1992: 366), 'many misunderstandings and ill feelings develop because of our different conceptualization of time lapse, the meaning of "punctuality", "tomorrow", "later" … or the need to plan ahead of time'.

Hall (1994: 266) differentiates between monochronic and polychronic time. Polychronic time 'stresses involvement of people and completion of transactions rather than adherence to present schedules. Appointments are not taken as seriously and, as consequence, are frequently broken'. Monochronic time 'is not inherent in man's biological rhythms or his creative drives'. Monochronics usually think in a linear fashion. For instance, monochronics schedule appointments linearly, arrival, meeting, conclusion, action, and they move through this same pattern all day long. When a monochronic is placed in a polychronic situation, stress and poor communication usually result.

Most Euro-Americans have a monochromic attitude toward time (Hall, 1984) and often prefer to do one thing at a time. They consider time as a valuable commodity that can be measured, saved, spent, wasted, bought and lost. How to get things done effectively is their primary concern, and the surrounding circumstances are not as important. In contrast, it is argued that black people do not schedule their time as strictly. They are satisfied with having a general guideline or plan and believe that everything has its own time (Akbar, 2004).

In the 'US [and Britain] promptness is highly prized … People make attributions regarding the person depending on how prompt or late that person is' (Brislin and Yoshida, 1994: 47). A large share of white peoples' relationships are governed by the clock. If black people arrive late for an appointment, they are labelled as being 'irresponsible', 'lazy', 'never on time'. Deviation from the set of rules people have learned in their culture regarding time 'tends to provoke strong emotional reactions' (Brislin and Yoshida, 1994: 47). This can result in interracial misunderstandings.

In African, African American and Asian culture, orientations to time are driven less by a need to 'get things done' and conform to external demands rather than by a sense of participation in events that create their own rhythm. African Americans 'often use what is referred to as BPT (black people's time) or hang loose time; maintaining that priority belongs to what is happening at that instant' (Samovar and Porter, 2006: 18). However, black people are capable of code switching with time. For example, the black professional may well be monochromic in the work setting, but polychronic in other settings, such as social and leisure activities.

Personal space

Hall (1955, 1964) was the first researcher to study personal space, systematically referring to the study of spatial usage as proxemic. Proxemics is a term that describes the study of the individual's use and perception of social and personal space. Personal space can be viewed 'as that area around each individual which is treated as a part of himself or herself' (Baron and Byrne, 1991). Barnlund suggests that 'Every individual, with guidance from his culture, also develops a sense of personal space, the distance at which he prefers to interact with others' (Barnlund, 1968: 515). It therefore follows that 'marked differences in spatial styles, then, may cause the same message uttered from various distances to be assigned different meetings and motives' (Barnlund, 1968: 516).

In a study of personal space among different cultural groups, Hall (1955, 1964) found that Germans used greater areas of personal space and were less flexible with their personal space than Americans. Arabs, French, and Latin Americans were more tolerant of sharing space and allowed much more flexibility than Americans. Close distances signal connectedness and bonding. In a number of studies, Halberstadt (1985) found that black Americans establish closer distances than European Americans. These closer distances begin in childhood when black American children establish closer distances in play and other activities (Aiello and Jones, 1971; Duncan, 1978). We should note that the nonverbal behaviours of touch and distance can signal involvement, connection, and intimacy.

In a study of middle class populations, Willis (1966) reported that African Americans greeted other African Americans at greater distance than whites greeted other whites. Moreover, whites greeted African Americans at further distances than they greeted other whites (Andrews and Majors, 2004).

The continued study of race and class proxemics could further enhance our cross-cultural understanding of black-white conflict and misunderstanding in every social institution, to say nothing of basis day-to-day 'spatial' interactions in social settings.

Facial expressions

The research carried out by Ekman (1972) on facial expressions in various cultural groups is useful. Ekman and Friesen (1967) argue that facial behaviours are both universal and culture-specific. According to Ekman, 'What is universal in facial expression of emotions is the particular set of facial muscular movements triggered when a given emotion is elicited' (in Harper *et al.*, 1978: 100). The authors note that facial expressions can also be culture-specific. Thus, because of cultural norms, individual expectations, etc., eliciting events for the same emotions can vary from person to person.

Implications for social workers

There are many occasions where misperception can occur in the contacts between white social workers and black clients, due to different display rules, different expectations, different attributions, etc. Social workers must show an understanding of differences between black and white groups – if these differences are ignored then the potential for misinterpretation will remain. A knowledge of the differences in white and black nonverbal behaviour has clear applications to social work practice. Social workers must be aware of the possibility that differences in nonverbal behaviour – both in terms of the kinds of behaviour carried out and how such behaviour is interpreted – may occur between whites and blacks. Although social workers must be aware of cultural differences in nonverbal behaviour they must be careful not to stereotype nonverbally the people from different cultures into cultural slots. It is important to note that not every black person will exhibit the nonverbal behaviours described above. While most of the work that has been done on the subject comes from the US, the results have clear implications for social workers in Britain.

Social workers in interracial communication must address themselves to the problem of overcoming the effects of strong racial stereotyping if effective communication is to occur. They must consciously monitor their attitudes and behaviours towards black people. Andrews & Majors (2004: 314) observes that 'the same behaviour performed by persons with different social characteristics or from different cultural backgrounds is likely to be interpreted as having different meanings'.

In an interesting US study of black-white interaction, Word *et al.*

(1974) found that [naive] white interviewers showed different patterns of verbal and nonverbal behaviour towards black as opposed to white job applicants (all applicants were confederates of the experimenters). The white interviewers sat further away from the black applicants, made more speech errors, and terminated the interview significantly sooner. The authors also found that when white subject-applicants were treated by white confederate-interviewers – as the black applicants were treated in the first experiment – they were judged by 'blind' raters to have been more nervous and to have performed less adequately than subjects treated like the whites. This study indicates that interviewer behaviours could mediate a self-fulfilling prophecy process by which the black applicants would wind up making a poor impression.

Social workers need to be aware of the 'conscious or unconscious racial stereotypes that [they] may hold and that will inevitably influence the treatment [interaction]' (Sanchez-Hucles, 2005). It is important that all social workers explore their own stereotypes (positive and negative) about black families (Sanchez-Hucles, 2005).

Social workers should be aware of their own attitudes and behaviour and those situations in which they are likely to display negative behaviours. Such awareness is at least a first step in mitigating problems in black and white nonverbal communication. Black people are 'very tuned in to nonverbals. For the social worker who has not adequately dealt with his or her own racism, the minority [black] client will be quick to assess such biases' (Sue, 2006: 167). For many white social workers, 'racism is a very painful topic, and they are likely to react negatively to it (Sue and Sue, 1994: 74). However, a worker who has not adequately dealt with his or her own biases and racist attitudes may unwittingly communicate them to his or her black client (Ridley, 1995, 2005). Indeed, the primary task of white social workers wishing to implement anti-racist practice is to change their own racist attitudes and practices' (Dominelli, 1997,40)

Finally, the literature that addresses impression formation from a black perspective is limited at best. If we are to appreciate and understand some of the factors involved in impression formation from a black perspective, much more research is needed.

3 The emergence of a black perspective in group work

Introduction

Texts on social psychology (e.g. Baron, Byrne and Branscombe, 2005) and psychology for social workers (e.g. Nicolson, Bayne and Owen, 2006) have had little, if anything, to say on the subject of a black perspective in group work. Descriptions of group process or climate issues related to race or culture have been infrequent in the literature (Helms, 1990), and, furthermore, recent publications intended to summarize the literature in, for example, group therapy (Stone, 1990) have not acknowledged the importance of race or ethnicity in group composition. Considerable attention has been given to the importance of race in one-to-one therapeutic practice (Kadushin, 1990, 1997; Dana, 1981; Green, J., 1982). Unfortunately, less attention has been given to its importance in group work. Group-work theory, practice, and research have been traditionally devoted to the development of universal conceptualizations which can supposedly guide all group practice (see Yalom, 2005, for detailed discussion of group theory and dynamics). This perspective has resulted in most researchers and practitioners ignoring the impact of member and leader ethnicity on group process and outcomes (Sattler, 1977; Davis, 1979, 1980).

This chapter provides an overview of the major issues to be considered in introducing a black perspective in group work. The development of a black perspective in group work is more advanced in the USA than in the UK.

The chapter will address some of the essential components of group work with black people. These include group composition issues, the salience of race, group norms, group leader's task, black self-identity issues, and implications for social workers undertaking group work. It is argued that a knowledge of racial dynamics is essential in group work with racially mixed groups. Although most of the research in this area was initiated in the USA by black and Asian-American psychologists, it is applicable to group work in the UK – as black groups in Britain also face racism and discrimination.

There is a low level of interest in group work as a method of social work, particularly in statutory agencies where it tends to be confined to a few specialist areas of work, such as the recruitment of foster parents and work with juvenile offenders (Mullender and Ward, 1985, 1991). Social workers use group-work methods in working with 'user groups', 'client groups', and 'special groups'. Group work is a good way of working with people 'who are isolated and may need collective support, who are disoriented and dislocated and may benefit from a group experience, and who are disadvantaged and oppressed and may seek collective strength' (Ahmad, 1990: 61). Nicolson, Bayne and Owen (2005) describe group work as:

> Social work in which one or more social workers is involved in professional practice with a group of probably more than four clients at the same time [but] the aims and objectives and the shared characteristics of the members, and the tasks they perform may vary greatly.
>
> (Nicolson, Bayne and Owen, 2005: 77)

Given that most individuals who practise group work are white, while many who are recipients of that treatment are black, the occurrence of racially heterogeneous groups is likely to be, and remain, commonplace. Hence, I have chosen to focus upon the white worker who is currently leading groups or contemplating beginning a group which contains black members. The general principles of group work discussed in this chapter apply to different models of group work; for example, social group work, therapeutic group work and self-help or support groups.

Group composition

The issue of group composition is very important as race and ethnicity play important roles in the group process and in the attainment of group goals. Unfortunately, literature in this area is lacking. It is important for social workers who are intending to do group work to first determine client racial preferences for their fellow group members or group leaders. The question for clients with respect to the racial composition of a particular group is whether they wish to be a member of a racially homogeneous group (a group composed of racially similar individuals) or a racially heterogeneous group (a group composed of one or more racially different others). Although this area of research has not received much attention, the available information suggests that the racial composition of a group may be of significant importance to clients. A racially heterogeneous group can reduce racial stereotypes and prejudice (Chen and Han, 2001). However, black people may feel more comfortable with discussing their problems in a homogeneous group (Tsui, 1997). The question regarding the composition of a group (i.e., racially and ethnically homogeneous or racially and ethnically heterogeneous) can also be answered by the stated purpose or goal of the group.

Little research has been done on the subject of racial balance in group work. Authors who have written on group work and group theory have had little or nothing to say regarding race as it pertains to group composition (Garvin, 1981; Konopka, 1983; Yalom, 2005). However, the group leader has to make the important decision of how many blacks and whites to include in a particular group. The proportion or number of members of different racial groups relative to each other may influence the character of the group. Moreno (1934) was one of the first researchers to address the phenomenon of racial ratios in small groups. He introduced the concept of 'racial saturation point': that is, the number of out-group members which an in-group would accept within its boundaries. Moreno maintained that both minority and majority group members have developed a racial saturation point for one another – due to past intergroup contacts. Therefore, at the racial saturation point, the group will express anxiety and aggression towards members of the out-group.

More recent researchers – for example, Brayboy (1974) – noted that whites are reluctant to become members of groups in which they are a minority. Other research indicates that black and white people may have different perceptions of what the racial balance of small groups ought to be (Davis, 1979). There is some evidence to suggest that whites tend to be most comfortable in racially heterogeneous groups when the proportion of whites to blacks is around 70 to 30 per cent, whereas blacks are most comfortable when the proportion is around 50 to 50 per cent (Davis, 1981). In an American study (Davis, 1979) white and black male college students were asked to compose groups of individuals from a hypothetical list of potential members. Results from the study indicate that blacks and whites do differ significantly in their preferences for the composition of these groups. Black people prefer groups that are 50 per cent black and 50 per cent white. Whites prefer groups that are 20 per cent black and 80 per cent white. The study also found that factors which increase intimacy in the group, such as a reduction in formality of the group or decrease in group size, may further increase black preferences for greater numbers of same-race group members.

Davis (1979) maintains that whites, because of their numerical dominance in society, feel themselves to be psychologically in the minority or outnumbered, if blacks are present in numbers greater than their societal proportions. He warns group leaders that the dynamics of their small groups may be affected by their racial compositions. Davis suggests that, because white persons are so consistently in the majority, placing them in groups where they are not may produce in them a psychological state he refers to as the psychological minority. Thus, even though whites may possess numerical dominance in the group, the presence of minorities in numbers greater than 10 to 20 per cent may be so physically novel – i.e. deviating so far from their prior interracial experiences – as to create concern for control and dominance of the group. Whites in this mental state are said to be psychologically outnumbered. Conversely, minorities in racial ratios greater than 10 to 20 per cent, because they are so characteristically outnumbered, may feel themselves to possess greater influence and power than their numbers would suggest. Minorities in this mental state are said to be in the psychological majority. Some authors have noted that 'the salience of a group member's race appears to increase as the intimacy of the group increases (Triandis and Davis, 1965; Davis, 1979)' (Davis, 1984: 103). In groups that were more intimate (i.e. informal rather than formal) and smaller, black subjects selected more same-race members. However, no such effects were found for white subjects (Davis, 1979). These findings suggest that, at least for black people, race of group members may be of greatest concern in small, intimate groups. It has been suggested that group members should not be put in groups in which they are the only one of that particular racial group, gender, or any other salient characteristic. A person will usually drop out of a group if he/she is the only representative of a racial group among the members. People need a built-in support system – whether a subgroup, other similar people or an alliance with a group leader of the same race. It will 'reduce the probability of scapegoating, and provide each member with a "second opinion" by which to more accurately assess his/her perception of social reality' (Davis, 1984: 103).

These studies suggest that group leaders may experience some difficulty in forming a racially heterogeneous group that is to the satisfaction of both blacks and whites, as differences in racial ratio preferences could lead to member dissatisfaction, discomfort, and possible withdrawal. Group leaders could address these issues openly and help members to adjust to the group composition. Davis (1979) has indicated that, in a racially heterogeneous group, 'members of both races may be inclined to offer more valid reports of their true feelings to someone of their own race ... [which] suggests that biracial leadership may be warranted' (Davis, 1979: 212).

One of the major problems of racially heterogeneous groups has been that these groups tend to be predominantly white, with very few black members. Consequently, black group members 'instead of gaining support and strength, instead of sharing common feelings and aspirations have found themselves even more isolated and sometimes in threatening situations' (Ahmad, 1990: 62). Even in those groups where there are equal numbers of blacks and whites, 'there may be different perceptions about common issues that are difficult or impossible to share; there may be group dynamics that undermine black members' experience and contributions, there may even be a clash of interests and priorities between black and white members' (Ahmad, 1990: 62).

Ahmad (1990) also notes that black women may be encouraged by social workers to join groups, such as 'mothers and toddlers groups' and 'women's groups', in which they feel uneasy and unwelcome. Consequently, these women drop out of the group and are labelled by social workers as 'not being group oriented, reluctant to join groups, [preferring] to stay at home, [and keeping] themselves to themselves .... These comments demonstrate a lack of understanding of the limitations of group work with Black clients in an environment of white dominance' (Ahmad, 1990: 62).

Black projects and black agencies are responding to deficiencies in existing services and are being set up 'to meet the needs of black service users, rather than continuing the pretense that predominantly white agencies, with ethnocentric policies, can offer an appropriately multicultural service' (Mullender and Ward, 1991: 34). A project called Ebony was first set up in 1983 for African-Caribbean and mixed parentage children living in white foster homes (Miller, 1985; Mullender and Miller, 1985). The general aims of the group were:

1   to give members a positive experience of black adults as role models,
2   to help the children begin to establish friendships with other young black people in a similar position to themselves,
3   to inform the children about the positive contributions that black people in the past and present have made to British society,
4   to develop their self-esteem through this experience,
5   to acquaint the black children ... with the realities of being black

– including racism and discrimination – and to help them develop skills in dealing with these.

(Mullender and Ward, 1991: 26)

The work carried out in the above group is similar to the individual identity work described in Chapter 5. The Ebony project also included a group for the transracial foster parents. This project demonstrates 'the potential for innovative group work practitioners to redress the failings of a past era when ethnicity was frequently simply ignored' (Mullender, 1991: 23). Mullender stresses the importance of group work: 'Individual work simply cannot match the powerful new learning that occurs when members join together in groups' (1991: 41). In the USA, group work has been effective with black delinquents (Cross, 1976) and black secondary school students (Gatz *et al.*, 1978) and recently with African American youth in the criminal justice system (Harvey, 2005). In an article entitled, 'Counselling blacks: a group approach', Shipp (1983) suggests that the 'group format is a good medium through which to treat many blacks, because it is consistent with aspects of black culture, such as the extended family, close sibling relationships, and strong familial ties' (Shipp, 1983: 110). He suggests that 'group therapies are more effective than individual therapies with Black clients … [which could be due to the] Black client's cultural propensity for group experiences (Jackson, 1980)' (Shipp, 1983: 110). In order to help black (American) clients, it is necessary for group workers to understand:

> Black [African-American] behaviour as it integrates with African ethos. Within this framework, specific values, attitudes, and behaviours express: 1. Cooperation between and among individuals 2. The collective responsibility of individuals to his or her group 3. The interdependence among individuals 4. The commonality of individuals.
>
> (Shipp, 1983: 109)

More recently, Harvey (2005) has also stated that an Afrocentric approach is needed to deal effectively with African American youth in the criminal justice system. The Afrocentric approach 'incorporates the individual, the family, and the community as an interconnected unit, so that any intervention must include interactions with all three entities' (Harvey, 2005: 241).

Black people who value interdependence can gain much from the power and strength of collective group feedback. In a cohesive group atmosphere, members can be very supportive of one another in patterns resembling the family situation. Like family members, they will work together to solve one another's problems (see Chapter 4). Other authors, however, have noted potential problems with treating black people in groups, including their reserve in dealing openly with feelings towards the group leader. Group treatment has been viewed as potentially less beneficial for Asian/Pacific Americans, because of their cultural reticence about being confrontative and competitive and their reluctance to interrupt others who are speaking (Chu and Sue, 1984). These problems arise when conflicts generated by cultural differences among ethnic minorities are not recognized and attended to early in the group experience. Such problems can result in premature termination among these minority groups.

Another factor that needs to be taken into account is the level of acculturation (see Chapter 5 for discussion of acculturation) among Asians in the group. There may be differences between first and second and third generation Asians (Robinson, 2003). Those individuals adopting an integration strategy may feel more at ease in a heterogeneous group than those adopting a separation strategy (Chen and Han, 2001).

Due to a number of reasons, which include linguistic difficulties and a reluctance to 'open up' in a group situation, doubt has also 'been cast on the possibility of using group-therapy techniques [with British Asians], but … [some authors argue that] it … [is] perfectly possible to apply the general concept of group dynamics with sensitivity to cultural concepts' (Bavington and Majid, 1986: 99).

Race as an issue is an important interpersonal factor and hence always has significance for both group members and leaders. A black perspective in group work must focus on the status and strengths of black people. The group leader needs to have a knowledge of black community norms, and group norms must specify that ethnic differences will not be translated as ethnic deficiencies. It is crucial that group-practice methods are made more ethnic-sensitive.

Salience of race

Interactions that do occur between black and white people are largely limited to superficial encounters. However, because of their minority numbers and status, blacks as a group have frequently had more exposure and contact with whites than whites have had with blacks. Consequently, it is probable that white group leaders and white members may experience more anxiety in racially mixed groups than will the blacks in those groups. The beginning phase of the racially hetero-geneous group may, therefore, be even more anxiety-arousing than the beginnings of most groups. The group leader must attempt to make the initial group meetings as enjoyable and non-anxiety-arousing as possible.

Most group leaders are not very successful in negotiating conflict around racial issues (Brayboy, 1971; Helms, 1990; Helms and Cook, 1999) due to a lack of knowledge, a lack of skills, and the fear of being direct. Davis noted:

> Perhaps one of the most important attributes that group leaders need to have is courage; they must be willing to take risks. In this situation, the risk involves raising what is essentially a taboo topic – the perceived difference in race. Merely suggesting that this topic be discussed may raise both eyebrows and anxiety levels.
>
> (Davis, 1981: 158)

A discussion of the group's racial composition will serve the follow-ing functions: introduce the topic; give individuals an opportunity to express any concerns they might have; and acknowledge the salience of race. Since race has played such a significant role in black people's lives, it is generally a topic of considerable importance to them. It has been observed that in racially heterogeneous groups of blacks and whites, blacks try to point out the salience of race as a factor affect-ing life events, while whites may simultaneously attempt to deny its influence (Brayboy, 1971; Fernando, 2002). If this occurs, it should be acknowledged by the group leader and discussed in the group. I wish to emphasize that race is always important, and to be 'colour blind' does great harm to the group process by 'relegating group member interac-tions to a superficial level' (Mullender and Ward, 1991).

As discussed in Chapter 7, social workers adopting a colour-blind ap-proach take the view that black people are like white people. Dominelli noted that social workers made the following remarks to her: 'Race is unimportant. Knowing them as people is'; 'I treat black people and white people the same. We are all members of the human race. There are no differences between people for me' (Dominelli, 1997: 36). A colour-blind approach is 'a denial, both of individual percep-tions in a racist society and ... the fact that race matters because of the way most – or all – societies function' (Fernando, 2002: 132). In a racially heterogeneous group, 'it is important that the group leader attend to potential cultural differences, stereotyping and biases, com-ing both from the leader and from among group members ... these issues should be addressed directly as soon as they come up' (Ringel, 2005: 188).

Social workers leading a racially heterogeneous group may be reluctant to introduce race as a topic for group discussion for fear of creating racial tension. However, by discussing issues of race there is a greater probability of relieving group tension and it also sanctions future discussions of race. If race and ethnicity are not properly considered and integrated, even well-planned group work will not be able to achieve its goal and, in some cases, may produce unintentional damage to its group members.

Group norms

Group norms give some degree of order and predictability to the functioning of the parts of a group. They consist of guidelines to behaviour, that is, value judgements about what should and should not be done, and how to maintain social relations (Shaw, 1981). The ability of a group to make norms and rules appropriate to its own needs and purposes is important for group effectiveness and the well-being of members. Norms are created relatively early in the life of a group and, once established, are difficult to change.

A group will typically adopt the norms of the majority of its members, and this phenomenon is also true for racial norms. Indeed, the majority will attempt to influence the minority towards the group norm. Helms (1990, 1995) suggested that the internalized normative trends adopted from other more powerful groups to which potential group members belong constitute a 'meta-zeitgeist', which in a white-dominated society is a norm of white superiority or other race inferiority. Discussion of this norm in the group may promote an understanding of these influences on the group.

The black client integrated into a traditional therapy group is faced with a formidable power structure – a collective of therapeutic and cultural norms that manifest themselves through the group process and yet are not conscious and are not, therefore, available to analysis. The group worker conducting a multi-racial or multi-ethnic group is faced with the enormous task of bringing such norms to group consciousness, and establishing a new set of norms that take cultural variables into account and unite, rather than separate, along cultural or racial lines. Paradoxically, normative centrality can only be achieved through consideration of the cultural and racial differences that divide peoples and, then, through their inclusion into the group process.

The group norms are white group norms that, in themselves, resist intrusion and disruption from minority cultures. In this regard, it would be naive to assume that a minority group member would not react negatively – on either a conscious or a subconscious level – to a majority of whites who all share common values and behaviour, and are trying to assimilate the black member into what they see as the therapeutic milieu.

We need to develop group norms that do not denigrate group members because of their ethnic backgrounds. Group norms must specify that ethnic differences would not be translated as ethnic deficiencies. Leong cites many examples of the cultural values of Asian Americans that conflict directly with group work. The cultural value of 'deferential behaviour and not drawing attention to oneself ... [is in conflict with] the group climate of open and free self-expression' (Leong, 1992: 219).

Group leader

As black groups that are minorities are also a minority in most groups, the group becomes a microcosm of the larger society. It follows that the power relationships among various (racial and ethnic) groups are re-enacted dynamically (Ringel, 2005; Tsui, 1997; Tsui and Schultz, 1988).

Group leaders may repress their own personal stereotypes and fail to work through them – since the issues of race and colour are emotionally loaded concerns in British society. This can have a negative impact on group work. Before starting work with a group of white and black clients, group leaders need to examine their own racial stereotypes and show an understanding of the power relationship between the minority and the majority group. Ultimately, the success of the group depends on the facility of the group leader in managing conflict.

Social workers leading groups which have black members should pay attention to group dynamics as they are affected by a group's racial composition. They should ensure that the attempts of black group members to participate in the group are not frustrated or ignored. In addition, group leaders should periodically assess the participation rate of each member. Black people may behave differently in groups depending upon whether the groups are racially heterogeneous or homogeneous (Katz and Benjamin, 1960; Katz and Greenbaum, 1963). In racially heterogeneous groups black members have been shown to participate in the group process to a lesser extent than might be expected. This lack of participation could be due to a general lack of trust, or to what Grier and Cobbs (1968) have referred to as 'healthy paranoia'. In order to establish a workable relationship with group members, a group leader must achieve a basis of trust (Chen and Han, 2001). The experiences of racism and discrimination which black people in Britain and the USA face may lead them to distrust white group members and leaders. Black group members may question the intentions of the group leader and the other members – thus, they may be uncertain as to whether the group leader has their best interests at heart. They may also note that the group leader and/or the other members are not cognizant of the social realities of black people. The group leader may be required to exert considerable effort to establish trust from black group members (Sue and Sue, 2003). As noted above, the first step is for the group leader to acknowledge the potential significance of race to the client. 'Leaders must also model appropriate behaviors of respect and acceptance of individual difference' (Hurdle, 1990: 67).

The lack of participation of black group members may also be due to the low social status attributed to them. White group members may hold limited expectations of black group members, which may result in a misperception of black behaviour. For example, Cheek (1976) has argued that equal participation of black group members may be perceived by whites as arrogant or aggressive behaviour. Furthermore, some white group members may attempt to frustrate the active participation of black group members in an effort to keep them in inferior roles, while others may ignore their contributions, considering them to be unimportant or insignificant to the group process. This behaviour will not only alienate black members, but will also delay group development by limiting group cohesion and trust. Social psychologists use the term 'group cohesiveness' to refer to the degree to which group members are attracted to each other and the group as a whole.

Individuals from Asian cultures who regard persons of authority highly may literally not speak in the group, unless specifically addressed by the leader (Chen and Han, 2001; Tsui, 1997). Hence, Asian-American group members 'may view the leader as an expert from whom they can seek advice, direction and problem solving' (Ringel, 2005: 185).

Furthermore, many Asian Americans prefer 'a structured, problem-focused, task-oriented approach to solving problems .... [This] makes the more ambiguous and open-ended approaches to group counseling quite alien and uncomfortable for many Asian Americans' (Leong, 1992: 223). White group leaders can fall into the trap of pathologizing the group behaviour of Asian Americans or other minority/black groups. According to Leong: 'Ethnocentrism is the phenomenon underlying much of the insensitivity to culturally different clients. It is based on a hierarchical view of values and assumes that one's value system is best or better than others' (Leong, 1992: 225). White group leaders need to question their Eurocentric assumptions and be flexible in their approach to working in groups that are racially heterogeneous. However, if group leaders persist in using a Eurocentric framework, a high drop-out rate among minority group members is to be expected (Ringel, 2005). For example, negative outcomes for Asian Americans who participate in group counselling is highly likely if 'the cultural values of Asian Americans which include verbal unassertiveness, low level of emotional and behavioral expressiveness, and reluctance to self-disclose to strangers [are not pathologized by white group leaders who] expect equal participation from them' (Leong, 1992: 227). Group leaders must become aware that taking a group member's unique culture into account is even more important than when an individual client is treated (Ringel, 2005). Cultural competence is an important aspect of the leadership role (Chen and Han, 2001). In order to be culturally competent, the group leader should be aware of his/her 'personal values and biases; [develop an] understanding of the world-view of culturally different clients, and develop appropriate intervention strategies (Lum, 1999)' (Ringel, 2005: 184).

A lack of awareness of the impact of ethnicity in group work may actually thwart the process and outcome of group work. Training group workers to be self-aware and to acquire knowledge and skills related to diversity issues is the key to effective group work.

Racial identity issues and communication patterns

Studies on racial identity development, as discussed in Chapter 5, have not yet been incorporated into the majority of social work group training courses. Several authors suggest using a stage model of racial identity development for both the group leader and group member to see if they are at the same stage of racial identity development (Leong, 1992; Tsui, 1997).

The theories of black racial identity (for example, Cross, 1971; Thomas, 1971) are relevant to group training. As noted in Chapter 5, these stage theories are progressive, characterized by early confusion and a poor sense of identity and by later ethnic acceptance and identity integration. The racial identity models provide a context in which social workers can gain an appreciation for, and empathic understanding of, a black client's frame of reference (how he or she interprets the world).

Black self-identity issues are likely to affect the response of black people to the group experience. They may influence black members' perceptions of the legitimacy of ethnically mixed groups and their leaders (Helms, 1990; Helms, 1995; Helms and Cook, 1999). Those lower in black consciousness (pre-encounter stage – see Cross's model in Chapter 5) may devalue a group leader who is black, while those very immersed (immersion-emersion stage – see Cross's model) in exploring their blackness may question the legitimacy of any white leaders and may contribute to anxiety-provoking interactions with whites (Helms, 1990; Helms and Cook, 1999; Tucker, 2002). Group leaders need to have an understanding of black identity development and its effects on the group process. For example, pro-black and anti-white attitudes of a black group member could be interpreted by the group leader as a stage in black identity development and not as a personalized attack.

A subject that has not been adequately researched is white racial identity development and its effects on the group process. Helms (1984) proposed a five-stage model of white racial identity development. Prior to this model, no theory existed to 'explain how Whites developed attitudes toward their racial-group membership (White) rather than their "ethnic" group (e.g., Greek, Italian, German, etc.)' (Carter and Helms, 1990: 105). Katz and Ivey argue that whites deny that they belong to a race and that certain prescribed attitudes and values are associated with belonging to the white race. The authors maintain that 'White people do not see themselves as White' (1977: 486). White people may not have a sense of what their whiteness means to them (D'Andrea and Daniels, 2001; Dovidio *et al.*, 2002). Katz (1985: 616) points out that 'it is easier for many Whites to identify and acknowledge the different cultures of minorities than accept their own racial identity'.

Helms' (1984, 1995) stages are: contact (characterized by a naive lack of awareness of racial differences); disintegration (the person is forced to acknowledge that he/she is white); reintegration ('the person becomes hostile toward Blacks and more positively biased toward his or her own racial group' (Helms, 1984: 156)); pseudoindependence (characterized by an intellectual acceptance of white responsibility for racism); immersion/emersion (the person searches for an understanding of the personal meaning of racism and the ways in which he or she benefits from white privilege) and autonomy (acceptance of racial differences and similarities, and 'actively seeks opportunities to involve herself or himself in cross-racial interactions because he or she values cultural diversity and is secure in his or her own racial identity' (Helms, 1984: 156). Helms (1993) argues that the development of a white racial identity model is important, as:

> White people are born the benefactors and beneficiaries of racism, although they may not be aware of their bequest. Nevertheless, because racism causes White people to deny, distort and repress

the realities of race relations in their environments, it has negative impacts in White people as well as having benefits. Therefore, for Whites to develop a healthy White racial identity in a racist society, Whites must become consciously aware of how racism works to their advantage and make a deliberate effort to abandon it in favor of positive nonracist definitions of Whiteness.

(Helms, 1993: 241)

Helms contends that, although 'issues of intergroup conflict have been studied extensively ... theoretical discussions of how individual characteristics combine to form a particular group climate when race is a potential issue are relatively rare' (Helms, 1990: 187). She extended racial identity theory to the group process by describing types of communication patterns that might exist in the group. According to Helms (1990, 1995), there are four communication patterns: parallel, crossed, progressive, and regressive. Helms suggested that a group member's role as a majority or minority group member acts interactively with racial identity stages to influence the group communication process. In a parallel group, both the leader and members share the same stages of identity. When the leader and group are racially heterogeneous, then parallel relationships involve pre-encounter/reintegration, internalization/autonomy, and perhaps encounter or disintegration stages. 'The common theme in parallel relationships is inertia ... [but] this inertia is less problematic the more advanced the participants' stages of identity are' (Helms, 1990: 200–1). Thus, group members or leaders in the internalization or autonomy stages might be inclined to respect each other as racially different and this respect could encourage growth and an eagerness to understand others' worldviews. A crossed pattern exists when the stages of identity between the group leader and subgroups (within the larger group) represent opposite worldviews. Group participants are unwilling to look outside their own worldview in order to gain an understanding of others' perspectives. Helms (1990) asserts that:

Crossed relationships tend to be contentious and combative .... For instance, the Internalized/Disintegration crossed relationship ... might be one in which the leader (or coalition) is attempting to avoid discomfort by ignoring racial issues or turning them into something else, while the other party is attempting to accentuate discomfort for the purpose of better self-understanding.

(Helms, 1990: 201)

A progressive pattern exists when the group leader's stage of racial identity development is at least one stage more advanced than the group participants' stage. The leader who runs this type of group may be the most successful at challenging as well as supporting group members' views and identities. This pattern is considered to be the most effective in 'promoting the longevity and functionality of groups' (Helms, 1990: 203). In a regressive pattern, group participants' stage of racial identity is more advanced than that of the group leader. Thus, group members might be at the internalization stage of development while the group leader might be at the pre-encounter stage. Consequently, high levels of conflict with the leader may develop, and the development of the group may stagnate. It appears that the crossed and regressive patterns are the most damaging to the group process.

Helms (1990, 1995) also suggested that the strength of these patterns may be affected by the perceptions of power in the group as determined by the numerical composition of the group. Thus, as noted earlier in this chapter, black members may feel in the 'psychological minority' when groups are less than evenly divided among black and white members, whereas whites may feel uncomfortable in groups with less than 70 per cent white membership (Davis, 1980). This too, may vary with individual white members' levels of ethnic consciousness (Helms, 1990, 1995).

Group leaders need to become aware of their racial identity development, as well as how these identity issues affect group members and group work (Chen and Han, 2001).

The value of studying interracial communication using racial identity development models is 'that such situations may be rendered less mysterious and thus, more manageable' (Helms, 1995: 196). If, for example, 'the potential participants [white group leader and black group member] are crossed with respect to "racial" identity, then it is foolhardy to expect them to make peace without a peacemaker who can acknowledge the "racial" identity concerns underlying the perspectives' (Helms, 1995: 196). An awareness of a black identity continuum will compel the group leader to acknowledge, rather than deny, race and colour.

Implications for social work practice

Most social workers who begin group practice with black people are probably ill-prepared to do so. The following guidelines, in addition to those indicated above, are offered to help the social worker in developing a black perspective in group work.

1 Group workers must be in touch with their own biases towards black people before beginning to work with a racially heterogeneous group. This calls for an honest appraisal of the way they have been conditioned to think of black people.

   Group workers should be aware of the possible feelings provoked by silent black clients. The silent client is not a new phenomenon, and group workers are trained to deal with them; however, if we add the variable of a different cultural/racial background, the group worker may feel quite bewildered. The following questions may be posed by the group leader: What does a silent presentation in this context mean, and how does this differ from the silence of a white client? Group workers need to anticipate their own reactions and those areas of bias that might contaminate their response. Such preparation will diminish potential areas of difficulty and allow the planning of appropriate interventions. In addition, group workers must be willing to work through similar issues with white group members and, most importantly, be able to serve as role models for all members. The workers' ability to stand firm, contain anxiety, and mould a group norm of openness, acceptance of individual difference, and willingness to integrate a variety of cultural experiences in the group process will counteract the tendency of the group to polarize along racial or cultural lines.

2 Group workers should encourage comments from group members about their perceptions of group work, i.e., what the group process is all about, and what they expect from the group process. Group workers should take an active role in generating a set of group norms which is by and large in keeping with the varying cultural backgrounds and personal expectations of the group members. They should also educate members of the group as to their function in the group, the behaviour expected, and the nature of members' relationships to the group worker and their peers. Norms that are evolved during this process can be periodically evaluated and modified as the group process evolves. Taking this crucial step in working with a racially heterogeneous group is imperative because it will put a stop to the natural tendency of the majority to define the issues and to shape the group process with their dominant cultural values.

3 It is often necessary to acknowledge and validate the unique life experience of black clients. Fernando argues that:

   Cultural sensitivity and the need to recognise and understand the social realities of the [black] clients' world [are important] ... but, if group therapists are open minded and sufficiently self-aware of their personal prejudices about race and culture, they could develop these attributes in the course of participating in multicultural groups.

(Fernando, 1988: 120)

Williams (2003: 727) notes that 'cultural competence has been reported as an important consideration in improving outcomes [in group treatment] for men of color'.

4 Group workers should avoid treating minority clients as representatives or spokespersons for their cultures or ethnic groups, and must assist other group members to avoid this pitfall. Treating them as representatives devalues their own unique life experience. A norm must be established in the group in which diversity is valued rather than ignored.

5 Group workers should become neither overprotective of the black client nor overly confrontative. Unnecessary protection of a client can arise from workers' projections of their own vulnerability or reactivation of their stereotype. For example, they may become overprotective of Asian clients, as they may assume that all Asians are nonverbal, helpless, and fragile. Such behaviour encourages other group members to treat the overprotected clients in the same manner or to ignore and devalue them. Excessive confrontation can result when the group worker becomes anxious, frustrated, or unable to draw the client into the group or establish any meaningful participation.

6 Groups should discuss stereotypes at all levels: personal, familial, and societal.

7 Confrontation is especially necessary when the group dynamics threaten to replicate the day-to-day oppression experienced by black group members. When issues of race, colour, etc. are discussed openly, the group becomes safer and a place where interaction and learning between black and white members can occur more easily.

8 Group workers must have ground rules about respecting other members – for example, 'non-acceptance of racist behaviour and gestures, non-entry of negative and offensive Black images' (Ahmad, 1990: 62). When white group members use racial slurs, one method for handling the situation is for the group leader to work with the group members both individually and in the group. The main challenge for the group worker is to create an environment that is safe and accepting enough to allow black and white people to interact in new and positive ways.

9   Group workers must be clear about their reasons for wanting black clients to join a group and the ways in which black clients may benefit from the group experience. It is, therefore, important for group workers to discuss these issues with black clients at the outset.

However, there may be many occasions when a racially heterogeneous group may not be appropriate for black clients. According to Sondhi:

This is partly due to the problem of communication and the inability to understand different cultural and social frames of reference. But it is mostly due to the fact that such projects have made most black people feel uneasy, if not unwelcome, since the most well-intentioned attempts at bringing people together were invariably set against the background of sustained hostility towards minority groups that made them cautious of any contact with white society and its institutions.

(Sondhi, 1982: 168–9)

A racially heterogeneous group can 'also result in increased anxiety concerning the exploration of ethnic issues [for black people]' (Ringel, 2005: 186). In such instances, white social workers should attempt to obtain information about the existence of black self-help groups, which are run by black people for black people. According to Ahmad:

Knowledge of these group work activities in black communities will not only widen the mainstream group work approaches, but also will enable group workers to use this knowledge to empower their black clients by giving them options and choices, through resourcing black group work initiatives and supporting them.

(Ahmad, 1990: 64)

Ringel (2005: 186) observes that a 'homogeneous group can become more cohesive and allow for more comfort with the exploration of problems ... [for] Asian immigrants'.

10   Group workers need to have an understanding of how black and white racial identity is formed, what factors influence its development, and what implications it may have for their work.

Conclusion

This chapter has identified some of the basic elements of group work with black people – from a black perspective. It is suggested that group leaders need to have knowledge of this information before attempting to lead a group which contains black members. Group leaders need to pay attention to the factors – a group's racial composition, the importance of race as an issue, the absence of trust, and the participation of black members in the group – which can influence the effectiveness of the group. Failure to recognize these issues can lead to structural division of the group along racial lines, to misinterpretation of the group process through unconscious defensive reactions (for example, reluctance to talk) among black group members and, probably, withdrawal from the group. These problems can be avoided if the group worker has a proper understanding of the dynamics of racially heterogeneous groups.

The success or failure of group work with black people includes many issues. Some of the more salient issues relate to race factors, images of black culture, racial identity factors, and the impact of the interaction among leader, members, and the black participants. Social workers engaged in group work with black people need to be cognizant of the issues addressed in this chapter in order to make sense of the behaviour of black group members.

Helms maintains that:

> Because Whites are the dominant race in [the USA], they can choose environments that permit them to remain fixated at a particular stage of racial consciousness .... Since Whites usually do have greater freedom to leave arenas in which their racial attitudes might be challenged, it is possible that each stage can culminate in either a positive or negative resolution. Positive resolutions should be associated with greater personal adjustment and better interpersonal relationships with people of other races.
>
> (Helms, 1984: 155)

4   The black family

Introduction

The traditional method of studying black families (in the social science literature) has often focused on the pathological rather than on the strengths of the black family (Bernard 2001).

Understanding family and individual dynamics within black communities is made more difficult by conflicting messages presented in the mainstream academic literature (Hayles *et al.*, 2004). Traditionally, black families were characterized by negative paradigms. Several well-known studies of African American family life described these families as being disorganized, lacking in intellectual firmament, and unable to promote proper socialization (Moynihan, 1965; Frazier, 1939).

According to Billingsley:

> There are four tendencies in the treatment of black families in social science scholarship. The first is the tendency to ignore black families altogether. The second is, when black families are considered to focus almost exclusively on the lowest-income group of black families .... The third is to ignore the majority of black stable families even among this lowest income group ... and to focus instead on the most unstable among these low income families. A fourth tendency, which is more bizarre than all the others, is the tendency on the part of social scientists to view the black, low income, unstable, problem-ridden family as the causal nexus for the difficulties their members experience in wider society.
>
> (Billingsley, 1968:15–22)

Myers (1982) proposed that the research and literature on the black family could be understood in the context of several themes. These included: poverty-acculturation; pathology; reactive-apology; black nationalist; and proactive revisionist. The poverty-acculturation theme refers to research which suggests that black families 'were more successful and healthier to the degree that they were successful in acculturating to the norms, values, and standards of white middle-class society [e.g. Frazier, 1939]' (Myers, 1982: 42). The pathology theme is built on the principles of the black matriarchy, emphasizing the consequences of poverty. Research in this area 'presented empirical evidence associating the degree of familial disorganization with personality, cognitive, and social deficits in ... [black] children [e.g. Moynihan, 1965; Rainwater, 1971]' (Myers, 1982: 43). The reactive-apology theme challenged the pathology view, and argued that black families 'were essentially the same as white families except for the experiences of racism, discrimination and poverty [e.g. Willie, 1970; Scanzoni, 1971]' (Myers, 1982: 43). The research and literature linked with the black nationalist perspective emphasized the strengths and competencies of black families, rather than the deficiencies and pathology. Thus, 'previous deficits (e.g. family structure) were redefined as strengths (e.g. the extended kinship support system) [e.g. Hill, 1972]' (Myers, 1982: 44). This approach also aimed to provide legitimacy and validation of the black culture, which was said to be unique and distinct from the white European norm. The proactive-revisionist strategy allowed the old questions regarding the black family to be 'restated and reconceptualized in a more precise and scientific fashion .... With this strategy, a more complex and a perhaps more realistic picture of ... [black] family life is emerging [e.g. McAdoo, 1978; 1979]' (Myers, 1982: 44). The first three themes fall 'into [the] category of black families studied using non-black interpretive and/or conceptual frameworks' (Nobles, 1978: 679).

The black family represents an area in which the use of traditional white psychological models leads us to an essentially inappropriate and unsound analysis. Much of the literature on families pertains to the European-American family. Researchers in the poverty/acculturation, pathology, and reactive-apology themes attempted to use white family norms as a standard of comparison for black families. I have already pointed out in an earlier chapter that it is difficult, if not impossible, to understand the lifestyles of black people using traditional theories developed by whites to explain whites (White, 1972, 2004). Several black researchers and scholars have argued that the existing theoretical and conceptual framework for the study of black families is ill-suited to the study of these families. These models distort and restrict our understanding of the complexity of the black family because they introduce ethnocentric biases and distortions into the analysis. We need to develop an alternative framework which 'will be consistent with the sociopolitical and psychocultural reality of black people' (Nobles, 1978: 680). Our ability to understand black reality is limited if the 'interpretative framework' for the analyses of that reality is based on assumptions associated with non-black reality (Boyd-Franklin *et al.*, 2001; Clark, 1972; McAdoo, 2002).

The field of child development research also lacks a black perspective and, where research exists, is based largely on white middle-class children, assumed to be (or defined as) normative and generic to all children. The behaviours and patterns of development in non-white children are then viewed comparatively against this 'norm' and defined as 'exceptions' or 'deviations from the norm'. Such deviations are then attributed either to the characteristics (i.e., deficiencies) of the individual, or to inadequacies and deprivations of the environment. By relying almost exclusively on direct or indirect comparisons as the major research paradigm in non-white research, the behaviour of black people is seen only through 'white glasses'. Therefore, by definition, black behaviour achieves the status of a legitimate scientific phenomenon only if it is evaluated from the perspective of the majority culture, and viewed against white norms and standards of behaviour.

Researchers of black families must guard against classifying the 'black family' as a single entity, rather than recognizing that, indeed, no 'one' description accurately characterizes the black family (Billingsley, 1968). One of the fundamental premises of Boyd-Franklin's (2003) book, *Black Families in Therapy*, is the recognition of cultural diversity among black families: 'Given the heterogeneity of cultural variables that are present in Black families and communities, it ought to be patently clear that there is no such entity as "the" Black family' (Boyd-Franklin, 2003: 6). However, she adds that 'While it is necessary to emphasize the heterogeneity of Black families, of equal importance is the consideration of how Black … families differ from other ethnic groups' (Boyd-Franklin, 2003: 7). The experience of black people in the USA has been distinct from that of other ethnic groups in four main areas: 'the African legacy, the history of slavery, racism and discrimination, and the victim system' (Boyd-Franklin, 2003: 7). While there are differences between the experiences of black people in Britain and in America, it is worth bearing the African-American experience in mind (see Chapter 1).

The issues discussed in this chapter are offered as the beginning steps towards an understanding of black family life. There is a tendency among social workers, based on the pejorative social science literature, to view the standard of white nuclear families as ideal, and to view the variety of family structures in the black community as pathological.

White social workers 'constantly belittle black families by pathologising them, seeing in them only weaknesses and ignoring their strengths' (Bernard, 2001; Dominelli, 1997: 94).

We need to free ourselves from the legacy of white research and begin to develop a black theoretical analysis of the black family. In this chapter, particular attention is given to the existing pathology-oriented black family literature, as well as discussion of the strength-oriented perspective on black family life. Strengths research continues today (Gadsden, 1999; Hayles *et al.*, 2004).The last part of this chapter discusses the implications for social work practice.

Negative images in the perception of black families

Early classic studies by DuBois (1908) and Frazier (1939) can be categorized in the first phase of poverty/acculturation. They were the first to focus on the black (Afro-American) family as a legitimate area of research activity. Central to their thinking was the notion that Afro-Americans were more successful and healthier to the degree that they were successful in adopting the norms, values, and standards of white middle-class society. Familial disorganization (i.e. Afro-American matriarchal structure) and pathology seen in lower class Afro-American families were described as products of slavery, racism, and poverty that established and reinforced lifestyles and patterns of behaviours unfavourable to effective acculturation. Emphasis in their research was on the detrimental effects of poverty and discrimination. Frazier maintained that as 'a result of the manner in which the Negro was enslaved, the Negro's African cultural heritage has had practically no effect on the evolution of his family in the United States' (1939: 66). The African-American middle class was presented as evidence of African-American familial stability, achievement, and success, due to its acculturative prowess.

Fortunately, more authentic perspectives have been offered that focused on strengths and resilient tendencies of African American families (Hill, 1972, 1999; McAdoo, 2002).

In a classic report, Hill (1972) identified five major strengths manifested within African American families: (1) adaptability of family roles; (2) strong kinship bonds; (3) strong work orientation; (4) strong religious orientation; and (5) strong achievement orientation.

Hill (1972) contends that 'most discussions of black families tend to focus on indicators of instability and weakness. With few exceptions, most social scientists continue to portray black families as disorganized, pathological and disintegrating' (1972: 37). Frazier's (1939) book, *The*

Negro Family in the United States, is considered to have established the 'pejorative tradition' in the study of black families in general and low-income black families in particular (Hill, 1972).

Frazier's line of research was followed by a number of investigators (for example, Moynihan, 1965; Rainwater, 1970), and resulted in proposals for social policy. In a document presented to the Office of Policy Planning and Research of the United States Department of Labour, Moynihan presented a devastating picture of black families: 'At the heart of the deterioration of the fabric of Negro society is the deterioration of the Negro Family …. It is the fundamental source of the weakness of the Negro Community at present' (1965: 15).

Moynihan presented empirical evidence associating the degree of familial disorganization with personality, cognitive, and social deficits in black children. Moynihan proposed the thesis that the deterioration of the black family was at the root of the deterioration of the black community. For the first time, the black family as victim became characterized as the agent of its own oppression. Moynihan saw the continual expansion of welfare programmes as a measure of the 'steady disintegration of the Negro family structure over the past generation' (1965: 6). He described black family life as a 'tangle of pathology' and considered these behaviours to be so much a part of black life that they became self-perpetuating, and therefore not needing white oppression or discrimination to perpetuate them. Moynihan regarded the black woman as perpetuating a matriarchal culture, which was in turn regarded as perpetuating pathology due to its nonconformity to the 'normal' family structures of the dominant culture. He argued that black women were too dominant, were more likely to find work, and were therefore too independent.

Pathology model and black families in Britain

This section will focus on the dominance of pathology models of black family functioning – with reference to models of African-Caribbean and Asian family structures in social science, and social work literature and practice. Barn (2002: 9) writes that: 'Negative thinking feeds into policy and practice, leading to discriminatory behaviour and poor outcomes for black families'.

Many social work texts paint crude cultural stereotypes of black families. The 'norm' against which black families are, implicitly or explicitly, judged is white. This norm presents a myth of the normal family as nuclear, middle class, and heterosexual. Black families are seen as strange, different, and inferior. The pathological approach to black family life is evident in the British research on black people. It is also evident in social workers' perception of black families. Social workers tend to rely on Eurocentric theory and practice, that devalues the strength of Black families (Ahmad, 1990; Graham, 2007).

In research carried out on social workers in London in 1983/84, Stubbs observed 'the ease with which negative models of Afro-Caribbean culture and family functioning, already prevalent within the social work literature ... fit into the frameworks of knowledge held by social workers to be relevant to their task' (Stubbs, 1988: 103).

It appears that little has changed since Moynihan's influential report on the 'Negro' family in the USA (1965) which defined the black family as pathological (i.e., family is inherently weak, unstable, and diseased). Lawrence argues that:

> the images about the Afro-Caribbean 'family' are similar to Moynihan's ideas about Afro-American 'matriarchal structures', the images of Asian family/kinship are ... different. Nevertheless the pathological approach to black family life which characterizes Moynihan's report is evident in British research on black people.
>
> (Lawrence, 1982: 117)

Ernest Cashmore, for example, argues that Afro-Caribbean youth gets involved with the British police due to 'the lack of social control exerted by the West Indian family, due historically to the fragmentation of family structure in slavery' (Cashmore, 1979: 139). Many social science and social work texts focus on:

> the weakness of the Afro-Caribbean family and this is traced to the absence of a stable father figure, so that families are seen as female-dominated or marked by a degree of instability in marital or common law unions. Problems of identity are said to arise from this instability.
>
> (Gambe *et al.*, 1992: 23)

In contrast to what is known about white families, little is known about black British families of Afro-Caribbean origin (Graham, 2007; Phoenix, 1988). The information available suggests that African-Caribbean families tend to be 'single parent' and that African-Caribbean mothers tend to be employed outside the home while their children are young. It is argued that:

these features ... produce many of the ills of the 'black community'. Thus the violence of West Indian (male) youth, the underachievement of West Indian children ... have all been attributed to the deviant family organisation of the West Indian family ... unsubstantiated beliefs that inadequate West Indian parents produce inadequate and delinquent West Indian youth permeate journalistic and academic discourses.

(Phoenix, 1988: 11–13)

Gambe *et al.* also point out that 'a great deal of sociological and social work literature makes reference to what it sees as endemic "intergenerational conflict", and the supposed involvement of Afro-Caribbean young people in many criminal activities' (1992: 24). They consider that 'the eradication of this perspective [pathology model], born out of Britain's imperial legacy, will take considerable efforts and action to achieve' (Gambe *et al.*, 1992: 24). The following quote from Stubbs' work illustrates the continued use by social workers of the pathology models:

Black teenagers coming into care, I think they have a fairly high profile in terms of strains becoming more apparent within black families which I think have to do with culture clashes in terms of more rigid ideas of their parents, perhaps, and behaviour of the teenage kids, and the tension that's resulted has triggered off the kids coming into care.

(Stubbs, 1988: 103)

In social science and social work literature, Asian families have also been described in terms of cultural stereotypes. It is the strength of Asian culture which is seen to be a source of both actual and potential weakness. Asian families are labelled as problematic, since their family structure is too tight and rigid. It is contended that Asian families are inclined to be insular since they seek to preserve religious and cultural traditions and extended family networks. Parmar points out that 'the traditional Asian household organised through the extended family kinship systems is held out to be responsible for a number of problems that Asians face in the context of British society' (1981: 21). It is argued that the 'rebellion' that 'Asian parents face from sons and daughters is ... to be expected and deserved particularly if they [Asian parents] insist on practising such "uncivilised" and "backward" customs as arranged marriages' (Parmar, 1981: 21). Young people, particularly young women, are said to be torn between two cultures (Anwar, 1998), unable to tolerate strict rules (in particular arranged marriages), and ill-equipped to integrate into British society. Complex family situations tend to be reduced to simplistic, catch-all explanations, such as 'endemic culture conflict' which offer no real understanding, and fail to give any positive regard to the client's cultural roots (Ahmed, 1986).

In the literature on Asian families in Britain, one can see that the key concepts within which the pathology of the Asian family is embodied are: identity crisis, cultural conflict, and language and communication problems (Lau, 2002). Discussions on cultural conflict, for instance, set Asian youth apart as a 'problem category' (Anwar, 1998; Ballard, 1979). The concept of cultural conflict 'assumes that cultural values are fixed and static and that there is no possibility of adaptation, flexibility or accommodation between one set of values and another' (Ballard, 1979: 109). However, existing research suggests that young Asians are no more alienated from their parents than any other group of young people. In fact, Ballard has indicated that 'only a small number of second generation Asians actually reject, or wish to reject, their families and communities completely' (Ballard, 1979: 110).

According to Small (1984: 279), the deficit model 'has entered social work practice as the conventional wisdom that guides the understanding of black families. It ... shapes the style of social work that is carried out with black families' (Small, 1984: 279). A discussion of second-generation Asians assumes that there are conflicts between them and their parents (Anwar, 1998; Lau, 2002). Consequently, social workers interpret the problems of Asian adolescents in terms of a 'culture conflict'. Implicit in the idea of 'culture conflict' is the assumption that the values of British family life are modern and superior while, the Asian culture is in some way backward and inferior.

Bernard (2001: 14) argues that 'by implicitly using the experiences of white nuclear middle class families as normative, the state reinforces a particular image of white middle class motherhood against which all mothers are judged, and in the process has pathologised black motherhood as deficient .... black people may not necessarily see professional helpers as protectors of their communities'.

Black family life researchers have focused on the 'problems' inherent in black family system. Past research concluded that 'the black family system was an organization inherently laden with problems and inadequacies' (Nobles, 1978: 679). However, this does not mean that black family life is free of 'problems'. Nobles argues that 'being black in a white, racist society is problematic by definition. Consequently, the family life of black people would be and is characterized by real and definite problems associated with racism and oppression' (Nobles,

1978: 679). Both racism and discrimination affect a black person throughout his/her life cycle and have an impact on every aspect of family life in Britain today.

The strengths of black families

Research throughout the 20th century has ranged from the race-based models of pathology, to the more recent cultural deficit models, to the models of strength and resilience (see Gadsen, 1999 for a comprehensive review).

The pathological perspective makes the implicit value judgement that black families constitute legitimate forms only insofar as their organization and functioning approximates or parallels that of the white middle-class families taken as the norm. This method of studying black families has been challenged by various authors. Foster (1983) contends that, in order to solve many of the problems that black families incur, it is important to understand their strengths. The focus of black family research in the USA has shifted from a pathological to a strength model (Mathias, 1978). This shift is characterized by: an examination of black families within a black cultural context (Hale, 1982; Nobles, 1978, 2004); a consideration of the role of grandmothers and other extended family members in child-rearing and child-development activities (Hale, 1982; Martin and Martin, 1978; Willie, 1982); and an analysis of the presence rather than the absence of the father within the family (Cazenave, 1979; McAdoo, 1981a, 1996, 2002). In Britain, as discussed earlier, the pathological approach to black family research persists. The pathological model fails to study the survival techniques used by black families in adverse situations (Bernard, 2001). In contrast, the strength approach takes into account those characteristics within the black cultural context that enable the black family to overcome adverse situations.

The studies which concentrated on the dysfunctional and disorganized aspects of black family life have been challenged by a number of US researchers (Billingsley, 1968; Hill, 1972, 1999; Staples, 1971; White, 1972, 1984). These authors challenged the (mainly) white researchers' preoccupation with pathology in the study of black family life. Implicit in the discussion of the deficit view of black family life is 'an assumption regarding normative model families. The belief that a statistical model of the ... family can be identified and used to ascertain the character of the families of all ... cultural groups is mythical at best' (Dodson, 1988: 81). However, as McAdoo points out:

The demythologization of negative images about the Black family is an ongoing process that will probably continue for generations, for the ethnocentric concepts held by the mainstream social science literature about black families will persist.

(McAdoo, 1996: 8)

Emphasis on strengths and competencies must replace attention to pathology and deficiency. Some researchers have been able to go beyond the negative stereotypical views that have been held on black families and have redefined previous deficits (e.g., family structure) as strengths (e.g., the extended kinship support system). 'Strengths' in this discussion denotes those characteristics of the family that enable it to meet the internal needs of family members, as well as those needs imposed by the external environment.

Studies on the strengths of black families began in the late 1960s, mainly in the USA. There is very little research on the black family in Britain, especially on black family strengths. Hill (1972) suggested that black families in the US utilize specific strengths in attempting to meet the needs of their members. Among other African-American researchers of the black family, there is virtually unanimous agreement that the characteristics that help black families to develop, survive, and improve are consistent with Hill's (1972) analysis of black family strengths. In a classic report, Hill (1972) lists the following strengths as characteristic of black families: strong kinship bonds, strong work orientation, adaptability of family roles, high achievement orientation, and strong religious orientation. Hill (1999) maintains these characteristics continue to operate as mechanisms for survival, advancement and stability. The work of McAdoo is one example of the scholarly contributions that support the description of the above-mentioned as strengths that are evident in the lives of African Americans. McAdoo (1992) conducted a study of the upward mobility patterns in middle income black families. She examined the extent to which upwardly mobile mothers maintained familial and cultural ties and benefited from their extended family network. Her findings revealed that the family served an important supportive function both emotionally and financially in their upward mobility. McAdoo (1995) examined the role of religiosity, levels of stress and family help patterns in middle and working class African American women and found that 94 per cent adhered to some form of religiosity. The women in this study considered religion to serve important functions to families and provided a system of beliefs. However, although the subjects reported being fairly religious, they had higher stress scores. Although these same subjects also reported infrequent church attendance, they reported the use of prayers and having faith as a coping strategy to deal with the effects of stress.

Strong achievement orientation continues to be a strength in black (African American) families. In McAdoo's (1992) study, the findings revealed that parents placed a premium on educational pursuits and pooled the resources of members of their extended family network to provide educational mobility for their children. Educational mobility was seen as a collective effort that included relatives and nonrelatives. This work endorses the cultural integrity inherent in the cultural values and practices of African American families.

Some of the prevailing strengths evident in black families have been summarized in Hayles *et al.* (2004): kinship networks and extended family systems; value systems that emphasize such things as harmony, cooperation, interdependence, acceptance of difference/diversity, internal development, strong work and achievement orientation, and traditionalism; strong male/female bonds; role adaptability and flexibility; roots, emotional support and buffers or consolations against racism; respect, appreciation, and full utilization of the skills and wisdom of senior family members; child centeredness.

McAdoo (1997) also describes cultural patterns that contribute to strengths and resiliency among black families. They include a supportive social network, flexible relationships within the family unit, a strong sense of religiosity, use of extended family, and the adoption of fictive kin. McAdoo (1997) cautions that although some commonalities exist, there is a great deal of diversity among black families. She also believes that 'some of the cultural patterns that have promoted resiliency have been eroded because of poor economic conditions'. Contemporary publications about black/African American families (Boyd-Franklin, 2004; Hayles *et al.*, 2004; Toliver, 1998) continue to reaffirm these strengths.

In a study of ethnic minority families in London, Hylton (1997) listed the following survival strategies of African and African Caribbean family survival strategies: 'spirituality; religion; holding alternative worldviews; maintaining the concept of 'family' as all blood relatives; focus on family and links with ethnic group; joint decision making (African Caribbeans); males as the main decision makers (Africans)'. Some of the key aspects of South Asian family survival strategies included: 'spirituality, focusing strongly on religion as a way of life, holding alternative worldviews, viewing families as the site of reciprocal arrangements of independence and dependence' (Hylton, 1997).

Black family strengths should not be viewed comparatively (i.e.

as perceived to be stronger than in other ethnic groups/cultures) but merely as inherent within the black cultural framework.

The extended family

Martin and Martin define the black extended family as follows:

> a multigenerational, interdependent kinship system which is welded together by a sense of obligation to relatives, is organized around a dominant figure; extends across geographic boundaries to connect family units to an extended family network; and has a built in mutual aid system for the welfare of its members and the maintenance of the family as a whole.
>
> (Martin and Martin, 1978: 1)

Hylton (1997) found that the term 'family' among ethnic minority families is seen as encompassing aunts, uncles, nieces, nephews and grandparents – what white British people call the extended family. Within the Pakistani community there is a strong emphasis on wide family groups that can include parents and married children with their spouses and children, also grandparents or in-laws (Hylton, 1997: 13). In Barn's (2006: 20) study of parenting in multiracial Britain, 'a quarter of the Asian parents in [the study] reported living with their own or their partner's parents ... compared to a small number of the white group'. Barn (2006: 20) found that 'whilst the wider [extended] family is important to minority groups, the process of migration from their countries of birth to Britain has resulted in the fragmentation of the wider family network for some ... [for example] the non-availability of grandparents'.

The black extended family, with its grandparents, biological partners, and other relatives, is an intergenerational group. One of the strengths that has been recognized in black families is that of strong kinship bonds and extended family relationships (Billingsley, 1968; Graham, 2007; Hill, 1972, 1999; McAdoo, 1981a; McAdoo and McAdoo, 1985; Parham and White, 1999; Stack, 1974; White, 1972, 1984). However, Hill points out that an 'emphasis on the strengths or the positive functions of the extended family [must not] obscure the fact that the extended family network may also have some negative or dysfunctional consequences' (1999: 38).

Parham and White (1999) discuss how cultural values and practices from traditional African families are seen among contemporary African Americans in their family practices. Values of interconnectedness, responsibility, and cooperation can be seen operating within African American families much as they operate in African families. Child rearing in African families is done by the extended family, and extended family members are also responsible for disciplining and punishing the child. Family members besides the biological parents socialize and discipline children.

Within the black family it has been quite common, for several generations, for parts of kinship groups to live under the same roof. These additional members very often are children and the elderly (Hill, 1972, 1977; McAdoo, 1981a). However, the absorption of whole families into the family unit has not been infrequent among black families. There are many different models of the black extended family (Billingsley, 1968; Hill, 1977, 1999; McAdoo, 1981a; White, 1984). Billingsley (1968) divides black extended families into four main parts: subfamilies; families with secondary members; augmented families; and 'nonblood relatives'. Subfamilies refers to families consisting of at least two or more related individuals. There are many examples of black extended families containing 'secondary members' (Hill, 1977). The majority of these family members are children.

The adult 'secondary members' fall into the following three categories: peers of the primary parents; elders of the primary parents; and parents of the primary parents. Augmented families refers to nonrelated friends living with the family. Nonblood relatives refers to individuals who are not related by blood ties but who are part of the 'family' in terms of involvement and function. Nobles (1974) has also noted that the black community is oriented primarily towards extended families, in that most black family structures involve a system of kinship ties. Nobles (1974) believes that in the USA the black kinship pattern was derived from African cultures not destroyed in slavery.

In a study of midwestern urban families in the USA, Hays and Mendel (1973) found that with the exception of parents, blacks interact with more of their kin than do whites. Black families also receive more help from kin and have a greater number and more diversified types of relatives living with them, than do white families. Stack (1974) has described in detail the reciprocity (i.e. the process of helping each other and exchanging and sharing support as well as goods and services) which exists in many black extended families. The reciprocal extended family help patterns continue even when black families have moved up the social class ladder (McAdoo, 1978, 1996).

Minority status in a hostile society tends to strengthen kinship ties (Hays and Mendel, 1973). Studies in the USA have shown that the extended family acts to preserve black family life (McAdoo, 1978;

Staples and Mirande, 1980). Ballard argues that, for Asian families in Britain, 'the concept of being part of a large kinship group, with its concomitant loyalties and obligations, remains very strong' (Ballard, 1979: 112) (see also Barn, 2006).

Another important indication of these kinship bonds is the system of informal adoption, which is prevalent in the black community. In the USA, original adoption agencies were not designed to meet the needs of black children (Billingsley and Giovannoni, 1970). Accordingly, the informal adoption process provided an unofficial social service network for black families and children. Informal adoption in black families (African-American) refers to an informal social service network that has been an integral part of the community since the days of slavery. It began as, and still is, a practice in African-American families to adopt the children of relatives and friends informally, and take care of them when their parents are unable to provide for their needs (Boyd-Franklin, 1989, 2003; Graham, 2007). These children 'retain their names as an important link to their lineage and kinship to their biological parents' (Graham, 2007: 84). This informal adoption network serves many vital functions for black families, such as 'income maintenance and day care, services to out-of-wedlock children and unwed mothers, foster care and adoption' (Hill, 1972: 3). In addition, it has served to strengthen kinship bonds.

Dominelli indicated that in Britain:

> Long-term fostering and adoption of children by others, particularly those who are closely connected with the children's original families, is a common pattern of childcare amongst people from West Africa (Ellis, 1972), the Asian subcontinent and the Caribbean.
>
> (Dominelli, 1997: 144)

Many black women choose to avoid the traditional policies and practices of adoption agencies and placement organizations and instead opt for adoption within the black community. Hill states:

> Since formal adoption agencies have historically not catered to non-whites, blacks have had to develop their own network for informal adoption of children. This informal adoption network among black families has functioned to tighten kinship bonds since many black women are reluctant to put their children up for adoption.
>
> (Hill, 1972: 6)

Close kinship ties have proven to be a major strength within black families. These strengths 'are … in need of support through imaginative adoption policies' (Hill, 1972: 8). Although social service policies in the USA have changed since Hill's report, and social workers explore extended family members as possibilities for placement, they often do not know enough about black cultural patterns to go far enough in searching for blood and nonblood supports. Consequently, as Hill (1977) has shown, black children are over-represented in foster care and residential homes.

There has been long-standing concern about the disproportionate number of black children in care (Barn, 2001; Barn *et al.*, 1997; NSPCC, 1999). Various authors (for example, Pennie and Best, 1990) have questioned the effectiveness of social workers in providing for the needs of black children. Pennie and Best argue that: 'Social Services should pay more attention to helping [black] families to develop family links and divert resources to reinforcing those links, rather than separating children from their families' (1990: 2). Parekh (2000: 185) observes that 'Asian and African Caribbean parents are the least likely to apply to the social services for help …'. Barn *et al.* (1997) found that 'training for [social work] staff and carers on equal opportunities and anti-racist practice was very sparse and lacked any impetus'. It is evident that social workers need to recognize the strengths of black families and they need to use black families in a positive way.

The proportion of extended Asian families living together is higher than among other groups, but this is not the norm (Modood *et al.*, 1997; Westwood and Bhachu, 1988). Although 'the trend … is towards nuclear families [it] does not mean that the importance of extended family ties has diminished. On the contrary, economic and material assistance as well as emotional support are found in these enduring links' (Westwood and Bhachu, 1988: 20). More recently, Hylton (1997) found that South Asian cultures 'limit independence by stressing mutual support and family ties organized around a strong religious and cultural base. Individuals are never truly independent because they cannot avoid responsibilities towards the extended family' (Hylton, 1997: 17).

In a book on the African-Caribbean family, Gopaul-McNicol (1993) indicates that:

> The West Indian family is usually an extended family that encompasses not only those related by marriage and blood, but also godparents, adopted children whose adoption is informal ('child lending'), and in some cases even friends. The function of these nonrelated family members is to provide security for children and to offer help in crises …. The extended family is a source of strength

for the couple ... [and] is particularly useful for women, who may rely on other women in the extended family for help with childrearing and household duties.

(Gopaul-McNicol, 1993: 22)

Lau (2002: 99) points out that 'the African Caribbean extended family functions by different rules compared with the extended families of Asian and Africa. Functional relationships are not necessarily defined by formal kinship'. In Asian extended families, 'individuation, personal autonomy and self-sufficiency take second place to interdependence and the need to preserve harmonious family relationships. This has led to the development of family structures that do not conform with Western European norms' (Lau, 1988: 279; see also Dwivedi, 2002). Similarly, African-American families show an interdependence or communal cooperation. In contrast, Euro-American families are more compatible with individualism and materialism (Foster, 1983; Robinson, 2001).

The rules governing intergenerational relationships in black and white families differ. For instance, let us consider the treatment of the elderly. In black (African-American) families the elderly are held in high esteem. Thus: 'Older women, more than men, are called upon to impart wisdom as well as to provide functional support to younger family members .... Children and adults are expected to show verbal and nonverbal "respect" to the elderly' (Hines *et al.*, 1992). The family elders are looked up to within the extended family network since they have the life experience that is highly valued in the black community. The hierarchy is clearly defined, with children being taught to respect their elders. For example, it is disrespectful for a child to call an adult by his or her first name. Children are expected to use titles, such as 'Mr' or 'Mrs', 'Aunt' or 'Uncle.' It is also considered impolite for a child to contradict an elder. Lau states that: 'The management of intergenerational conflict in these [extended] families must take account of the linear authority patterns, as well as important key relationships with a protective and buffering function not found in Western European nuclear families' (Lau, 1988: 280).

White social workers are more likely to tolerate intergenerational conflict between parents and adolescents in white homes than in black homes. Such behaviour is defined as 'culture conflict' in black families. However, the little research that exists suggests that young Asians, for example, are no more alienated from their parents than any other group of young people (Anwar, 1998; Westwood and Bhachu, 1988).

Another strength that has been recognized in black families is that of strong work orientation. Contrary to popular opinion, black families place heavy emphasis on work and ambition (Hill, 1972, 1999; Lewis and Looney, 1983). As 'families headed by women comprise the majority of families receiving public assistance, it is commonly believed that dependency is characteristic of most of these families' (Hill, 1972: 9). However, the majority of such families are not 'completely dependent on welfare' (Hill, 1972: 9). Unemployment statistics and benefit claims are usually cited as examples of the lack of a strong work orientation in black families. Little consideration has been given to the reality of job discrimination. For instance, in Britain, black people (particularly men) are more likely than their white counterparts to be unemployed. When they do work it is likely to be in the most menial and poorly paid jobs (Brown, 1984; Hare and Hare, 1984; Modood *et al.*, 1997; Parekh, 2000). There is a tendency to label black people as 'unmotivated' or 'chronically unemployed' – thus blaming them for the economic and social situation that has created their victimization. Social science literature has tended to ignore the stable black families in which hard work is an attribute (Hill, 1972, 1999; Lewis and Looney, 1983).

The fact that blacks must often work at the most menial jobs, receive less pay for comparable work, and often are the last hired and the first fired, gives credence to the assertion that blacks put forth much effort to be a part of the work-force. The working wife/mother is also a not-uncommon phenomenon in the black family, regardless of whether one or two parents are present (Billingsley, 1968; Hill, 1972, 1999; McAdoo, 1981a; Phoenix, 1988).

The role adaptability of black family members is another strength that is often overlooked in the Eurocentric social science literature. Freeman (1990) suggests that much of the role flexibility in black families developed in response to adverse external conditions. Due to the economic realities faced by many black families, this role flexibility developed as a survival mechanism. Older children often 'fill in' as parents for younger sisters and brothers while parents work. 'Black women have sometimes had to act as the "father" and black men as the "mother"' (Boyd-Franklin, 2003: 64). An example of fluid roles in the African-American family also includes extended family members and nonrelatives who share in providing emotional nurturance and carrying out instrumental tasks. Hill believes that 'such role flexibility helps to stabilize the family' (1972: 17). White notes that:

> a variety of adults and older children participate in the rearing of any one black child. Furthermore, in the process of childrearing, these several adults plus older brothers and sisters make up a kind

of extended family who interchange roles, jobs, and family functions in such a way that the child does not learn an extremely rigid distinction of male and female roles.

(White, 2004: 12)

The role adaptability of the single-parent African-Caribbean mother also needs to be recognized as a measure of strength. The assumption is often made that the one-parent family is inherently unstable; indeed, using the nuclear family as a model, one-parent families are often referred to as nonfamilies. But a major strength of black families is the ability to assume different roles as needed. Lau suggests that:

In conditions where West Indian men have felt demoralized, West Indian women have to assume a strong role as an adaptive response. She has had to compensate for the undermining of the father/husband role, due to lack of education, unemployment and inability to protect his family.

(Lau, 1988: 281)

Graham (2007: 85) points out that 'the positive attempts of black fathers to rear their children have received little attention .... the deviant behaviour of black men is a widely held perception in the wider society'.

Many studies of low-income black families fail to note strong achievement orientation. Hill (1972) suggests that in black families the desire to move from a position of disadvantage to one of advantage is a strong one. Black parents stress this factor to their children not only through verbal urgings towards success, but through behaviour to ensure the probability of achievement. In a study of well-functioning working-class black families, Lewis and Looney (1983) found that these families gave messages to their children such as that they could 'make it' in spite of discrimination. Many black families view education as a way out of poverty. Hill states that 'these strengths need to be built upon by truly making education the avenue for success' (1972: 32). Black families 'place great value on education and knowledge as a way of counteracting the effects of oppression and discrimination' (Graham, 2007: 84). This can be seen in the use of Saturday schools in black communities. In a recent study, Barn (2006: 3) found that:

black and Asian parents place an enormous importance on the value of education, and express a great deal of concern about the future of their children. The reality and impact of racism in their own lives and in the lives of their children was not far from the minds of minority ethnic parents. Good education was regarded as of the utmost importance to combat racial discrimination and disadvantage and to prevent social exclusion.

Another strength that has been widely discussed in the literature, but less frequently studied, is that of religious orientation. Religion was a primary component of family stability for the ancestors of American blacks, and spiritual beliefs have become a part of the survival system of African-American people. Individuals who grew up in a 'traditional black community' are equipped with a system of core beliefs, particularly spiritual ones (Mitchell and Lewter, 1986). This system of core beliefs is the foundation of the inner strength of the person.

Nobles describes the essential nature of African religious experience, noting the extent of the unified quality of the African spiritual sensibility:

> Curiously enough, many African languages did not have a word for religion as such. Religion was such an integral part of man's existence that it and he were inseparable. Religion accompanied the individual from conception to long after his physical death.
>
> (Nobles, 1980: 25)

The legacy of this belief system has survived years of slavery and has influenced both the strong sense of 'family' (i.e. the extended family group) and the very strong religious or spiritual orientation of many black Afro-American families today (Nobles, 1980).

Today, the church and the black family structure are interlocked and interdependent. The church for many blacks has traditionally been a refuge in a hostile world. It is a source of strength and hope for its members, and it gives them a sense of community. Even though the church is declining in importance, it still remains the single most unifying organization for blacks. Many authors have discussed the strong religious orientation of black families (Hill, 1972, 1999; McAdoo, 1981a; Pipes, 1981).

In their study of well-functioning working-class black families, Lewis and Looney (1983) found that a strong religious orientation was an extremely important value. Gopaul-McNicol notes that 'in the West Indian communities of the United Kingdom, religion plays a significant role in the social and political life of the people' (1993: 70).

The most controversial issue in the black family literature is the notion of the black family as essentially a matriarchal family. As mentioned previously, a number of authors (White, 1972; Hill, 1972, 1999;

McAdoo, 1981a) have challenged Moynihan's (1965) characterization of black families as 'a tangle of pathology'. He viewed the black woman as perpetuating a matriarchal culture – a culture that was in turn viewed as perpetuating pathology due to its nonconformity to the 'normal' family structures of the dominant culture. As noted above, the poor educational achievement of black (African-Caribbean) children is frequently blamed on 'father absence' (Swann, 1985). Similarly, 'analyses of urban unrest in the popular media give explanations in terms of the pathology of the West Indian family (Lawrence, 1982)' (Phoenix, 1997: 65). A number of authors (for example, Henshall and McGuire, 1986; Archer and Lloyd, 1982) have criticized research in this area.

Phoenix states that:

> For a variety of socio-political and historical reasons (including the fact that there are many more black women and black men in the USA) black women of Afro-Caribbean origin in this country, and of African origin in the USA are much more likely not to live with their children's fathers (see Bryan *et al.*, 1985, for discussion of the British situation, and hooks, 1982; Davis, 1981; see Marable, 1983 for the USA).

> (Phoenix, 1997: 65)

Recent data indicates that 48 per cent of African American children live in households with a single mother, whereas 16 per cent of white children live with a single mother. African American children are also more likely to reside in a home where a grandparent (s) is present than are white children (US Census, 2002). In Britain, a higher percentage of African-Caribbean households, compared with white and Asian households, consist of a single parent with children under 16 (Modood *et al.*, 1997). It should be pointed out, however, that the majority of African-Caribbean households with children do contain two parents. The proportion of single African-Caribbean parents is high only in comparison with the proportion of white and Asian single parents. The single-parent African-Caribbean mother 'has traditionally used many supports external to the family, including godmothers, neighbourhood networks and the Church' (Lau, 1988: 281).

The issue is not who heads the family, but rather the functionality of the family members present. The problems associated with poverty-level, female-headed families (poor jobs, education, housing, health care) can usually be attributed to economic deprivation rather than to the fact that the family is headed by a woman (Barn, 2006).

In a study of parenting in multi-racial Britain, Barn (2006) found that many of the Caribbean families experiencing financial and housing problems were lone mothers. Barn (2006) also found that low income, unemployment, and poor housing were characteristic of black, Pakistani and Bangladeshi families.

White (1972, 1984, 2004) contends that the black family is observed from a white middle-class perspective, 'which assumes that the psychologically healthy family contains two parents, one male and one female, who remain with the child until he or she becomes a young adult' (White, 1972: 44). As black men are often not 'consistently visible to the white observer' erroneous conclusions about matriarchy are often drawn. The matriarchal perspective has also been criticized for failing to take into account 'the extended nature of the black family' (White, 1972).

It is argued that the discussions of family stability that focus only on the roles of husband and wife or father and mother overlook the stability and support that have been provided by the extended family in female-headed households. If the extended family model is a more accurate description of the black family than the matriarchal model, social scientists need 'to move toward ways of strengthening the extended family, as opposed to some basic reorganization of the black family' (White, 1972: 45).

Social scientists need to move away from the pathological approach of much of the research on black families towards a black perspective that recognizes the strengths of black families.

Racial socialization

This section will focus on parental communications to children about race, a process researchers commonly refer to as 'racial socialization'. Racial socialization is defined by Peters (1985) as the 'tasks Black parents share with all parents – providing for and raising children ... but include the responsibility of raising physically and emotionally healthy children who are Black in a society in which being Black has negative connotations' (1985: 161).

Thornton *et al.* (1990: 401) defined racial socialization as including 'specific messages and practices that are relevant to and provide information concerning the nature of race status'. They further specified three realms of relevant information that parents may communicate: (a) information related to personal and group identity, (b) information related to intergroup and interindividual relationships, and (c) information on group position in the social hierarchy. Other conceptualizations have incorporated aspects of these definitions, focusing on the transmission of cultural practices, racial knowledge, and awareness of racism through verbal, nonverbal, deliberate, and inadvertent mechanisms (Bowman and Howard, 1985; Marshall, 1995; Sanders Thompson, 1994; Stevenson, 1994, 1995). Thus, the term refers to parental practices that communicate messages about race or ethnicity to children. It is applicable across multiple racial/ethnic groups. Johnson *et al.* (2003: 19) argues that 'racial socialization, preparation for the experience of ethnic or racial bias [is an important] component of parenting'. McAdoo (2002) referred to racial socialization as one of the most important parenting tasks of black parents.

The concept that black families have a special role in buffering the impact of racism and promoting a sense of cultural pride for their children has received significant attention over the last decade (Stevenson *et al.*, 2004). Many studies have attempted to define, measure, and promote racial or ethnic socialization for black children and adolescents. Demo and Hughes (1990) found that adults who had received racism preparation messages from parents while growing up were more likely to have stronger feelings or closeness to other blacks, and to hold stronger support for black separatism. Other researchers found a clear sense of and communication about one's racial identity from family members contributed to academic, and career success (Bowman and Howard, 1985; Edwards and Polite, 1992).

Stevenson (1998) and Stevenson *et al.* (2004) suggest that racial socialization messages may be proactive or protective. That is, they may originate from parents' preconceived values, goals, and agendas (proactive) or they may occur in reaction to discrete events in parent's or children's lives (reactive). Proactive racial socialization is linked to parents' views of the strengths and competencies their children will need in order to function effectively in their adult social roles. Proactive racial socialization among black parents is guided by parents' expectations that their children will inevitably encounter racism and discrimination (e.g. Essed, 1990). However, other racial socialization agendas also may be proactive. For example, parents who value diversity and pluralism may choose racially, ethnically diverse versus homogeneous settings for their children. An important feature of proactive racial socialization messages is that they are closely linked to parents' worldviews.

Reactive racial socialization occurs inadvertently in response to race-related incidents that parents or children have experienced, or in response to children's general queries about racial issues. Children can disagree with parents' socialization messages, choosing instead to stick to their own worldviews. Uba (1994) cites a case of conflict between a 17-year-old Korean American boy and his immigrant parents, which illustrates the ways in which children may choose to incorporate or ignore parents' racial socialization efforts. Uba states: 'Although his parents tried to teach him to be proud to be Korean and to learn about Korean culture, Jack did not identify with Koreans as much as his parents wanted. Jack's father had threatened to disown him for being so disrespectful and attributed Jack's behaviours to being too Americanized' (Uba, 1994: 113).

The different dimensions of racial socialization include: emphasizing racial and ethnic pride, traditions, and history (termed cultural socialization); b) promoting an awareness of racial prejudice and discrimination (termed preparation for bias); c) issuing cautions and warnings about other racial and ethnic groups, or about intergroup relations (termed promotion of mistrust); and d) emphasizing the need to appreciate all racial and ethnic groups (termed egalitarianism) (Boykin and Toms, 1985; Thornton *et al.*, 1990; Demo and Hughes, 1990; Sanders Thompson, 1994). Although dimensions of racial socialization are described separately, particular racial socialization messages as they occur in everyday conversation are less readily distinguishable. For example, messages emphasizing cultural pride and history (cultural socialization) also may contain messages about historical discrimination and prejudice (preparation for bias), at least among minority populations in the US and Britain.

Studies have also found that the majority of African American adults' recall receiving messages about race from their parents (Sanders Thompson, 1994; Demo and Hughes, 1990). (Garcia Coll *et al.*, 1995; Garcia Coll and Magnuson, 1997; Kibria, 1997). However, Boyd-Franklin (2003: 35) observes that some 'African American parents, particularly those who had achieved high levels of education and socio-economic status, began to feel that there was no longer a need to prepare their children for the realities of racism. Unfortunately, this often left their children defenseless against the entrenched, but often subtle, forms of racism that continues to exist today and led to serious damage to their self-esteem. These children are often referred to [clinical psychologists] for treatment'. These findings are relevant to the UK context (e.g., Banks, 2002; Maxime, 1993, 1997).

In Britain an important part of ethnic minority parenting is to teach children to cope with racism, prejudice, and discrimination. There is considerable evidence that there is discrimination against Asians and African Caribbeans in education, employment, the health care system, and law, including the criminal justice system (Brown, 1984; Modood *et al.*, 1997; Parekh, 2000). Indeed, racial violence and racial abuse appear to be on the increase in Britain (MacPherson, 1999; Skellington and Morris, 1992). Barn (2006) suggests that 'the task of ethnic and racial socializing is a challenging but important one for minority [black] parents and children. In addition, to creating a positive, nurturing and supportive environment, minority parents have additional tasks of giving positive messages about difference and diversity and to develop a sense of belonging'.

Racial socialization is an area that has not received much attention in the consideration of parenting in black families in Britain. Although most of the literature concentrates on African American parents and to a lesser extent Latino and Asian parents (Garcia Coll *et al.*, 1995; Garcia Coll and Magnuson, 1997; Kibria, 1997), we can posit that the processes may be similar in other ethnic and racial groups that are considered minority groups in Britain.

Very little is known in Britain about how the racial/cultural socialization process is carried out in different ethnic and minority groups. In Britain, Fatimilihein (2002) found that racial socialization influenced the racial and ethnic identity development of African Caribbean adolescents. She notes that 'racial socialisation messages relating to black culture and history, racism, pride, and the family [influenced racial and ethnic] development' (Fatimilihein, 2002: 355). There was also a strong relationship between 'receiving messages about racism [and] being more immersed in a black racial identity' [and concludes that] 'racial socialization has a major impact on racial and ethnic identity development' (Fatimilihein, 2002: 355).

Rodriguez *et al.* argue that 'By avoiding any conversations about race or ethnicity or ignoring situations that arise, adults may unintentionally send a subtle message that race or ethnicity is unimportant or not to be discussed openly' (2003: 3012).

Reynolds (2000) notes that an important mothering function of African Caribbean mothers living in Britain is to provide children with strategies to cope with racism. Reynolds notes that 'As a result of particular concerns facing African Caribbean young males ... in educational underachievement, schools exclusion, police harassment and incarceration, racial violence ... [it is important for parents to provide] them with the necessary guidance and advice to resist systems of racism and inequalities' (2000: 144).

In a study of Punjabi families in Britain, Dosanjh and Ghuman found that over 50 per cent of the Punjabi mothers in their sample 'said that they talk to their child about racism in general, and how to cope with the racism which they are likely to meet in their daily lives' (1996: 132). For example, one mother described her son's first encounter with racism: 'He had a few people say to him Paki. And he said to me: "Mum, am I a Paki". I said: "No, you are not a Paki". I went to his school and saw his teacher and told him: "he is not a Paki; he is a Sikh"'(1996: 132–3). In a study of permanent family placement for children of minority ethnic origin in Britain, Thoburn *et al.* found that young people's comments 'about growing up as a member of a minority ethnic group in Britain were often linked with comments about racism' (2000: 133). Most of the young people in the study 'felt that their adoptive or foster parents, whether of the same or a different ethnic background had been helpful [in helping them cope with racism]' (2000: 133). For the young minority ethnic people in their sample, good parenting 'must include help to deal with racism and with issues of identity and racial pride'(Thoburn *et al.*, 2000: 208).

Racial socialization and racial identity

The approach parents take with regard to the racial socialization of their children is often closely related to their own level of racial identity (McAdoo, 2002) (see Chapter 5 for discussion of racial identity).

Parham and Williams (1993) examined the impact of race-specific messages on racial identity attitudes. Participants were classified into one of six groups based on self-reported messages they received from parents regarding race. In that study, none of the four subscales of the Racial Identity Attitude Scale (see Cross, 1991 for details of the Scale) was found to be uniquely related to the parental messages received while growing up. There was no significant relationship between the set of four racial identity attitudes and six racial message categories. Parham and Williams (1993) stated that it was likely that their question on racial messages was not sensitive enough to detect a relationship between parental racial socialization and racial identity attitudes. It should also be noted that Demo and Hughes (1990) found a relationship between the impact of parental racial socialization on dimensions of racial identification, rather than attitudes associated with the racial identity stage. This may account for the difference in their findings. Thompson *et al.* (2000) also found a positive relationship between aspects of racial socialization and positive racial identity attitudes.

Demo and Hughes (1990), using data from the National Black Survey (US) reported a relationship between parental socialization messages and racial identity. They assessed black identity in three ways: feelings of closeness to other blacks, commitment to African culture and the extent to which blacks should confine their social relationships to other blacks, and the evaluation of blacks as a group. Parental socialization messages assessed what individuals had been taught about what it is to be black, and about getting along with whites. When 'feelings of closeness to other blacks' and commitment to black separatism were examined, parental racial socialization was one of the strongest correlates. Blacks who were told to view 'all races as equal' identified more closely with black people, their history, and their culture than did blacks who were told to 'work hard' or to view 'whites as superior'. The individualistic 'work hard' approach was weakly but positively related to black group evaluation. Demo and Hughes (1990) noted that their findings also supported a multidimensional approach to the study of racial identity.

Spencer (1983) found that children with some knowledge of black history as reported by parents were more likely to report black/Afrocentric racial attitudes, while children who were limited in knowledge about civil rights, who had parents who did not discuss race discrimination issues or teach about civil rights were more likely to report Eurocentric racial attitudes. She also found that young children (3–6 years) in general tended to hold Eurocentric racial attitudes but as they got older (7–9 years), an orientation toward Afrocentric racial attitudes increased. This finding was true irrespective of geographic region. In the study, Spencer asked parents rather than youth about their cultural values transmission.

In uncovering the various culture child-rearing strategies and messages identified by the parents in her different geographic samples, Spencer (1983) noted several themes. Those themes include parental teaching of the importance of civil rights, that integration leads to greater experiences, that the current racial climate is better than the 1950s or 1960s, and that racial discrimination exists. Parent and children's knowledge of black history was found to be correlated with children's pro-black racial awareness, racial attitudes, and racial preferences. Direct and active teaching from parents about cultural values is most crucial for instilling Afrocentric or pro-black thought processes in children. That is, without direct intervention, black children's pro-black identities may be subject to confusion and instability.

To conclude:

> Children and adolescents who are socialized about race and ethnicity are further along in identity than children who are not (Knight *et al.* 1993; Marshall 1995) and they demonstrate more positive mental health outcomes and competencies (Parham and Helms 1985; Phinney and Chavira 1995; Pyant and Yanico 1991; Taub and McEwen 1992).
>
> (Rodriguez *et al.*, 2003: 302)

Implications for social work practice

In general, social work has operated within a 'problem oriented' framework, which is characterized by deficit and dysfunctional theories of black families. Dominelli argues that:

> Black children and families are overrepresented in the controlling aspects of social work and underrepresented in the welfare aspects of social work .... We need a shift from a deficit model of social work control to a strength model of social work empowerment.
>
> (Dominelli, 1992: 166)

Social work models have tended to pathologize black families and encourage practitioners to perceive the families as being the 'problem'. Consequently, social work interventions focus almost exclusively on clients' weaknesses, inabilities, and inadequacies. The negative perceptions and assumptions about black families, and lack of understanding, awareness, and knowledge of black experience, become pervasive forces within social work that can endanger the welfare of black families. Traditional social work is not effective in meeting the needs of black families. A lack of knowledge of black families has contributed 'to unnecessary intervention of social workers in black families which often results in devastating consequences for the family' (ABSWAP, 1983: 14).

More recently Barn (2002: 12) observes that 'the extent to which education and training equip students in the helping professions to develop their skill and competence in engaging black families is questionable (Penketh, 2000)'. It is important that all social workers 'develop their skill and competence in working with minority ethnic birth and substitute families' (Barn, 2002: 12). A strengths-based approach calls for looking at individuals, families, and communities in the light of 'their capacities, talents, competencies, possibilities, visions, values, and hopes, however dashed and distorted these may become through circumstance, oppression and trauma' (Fong, 2004: 136).

Social workers must recognize that culture is never static and black families must not be judged on the basis of cultural preconceptions. They need to assess black families in the context of a racist society, and mobilize the strengths and competence in black families. Most black researchers agree that the characteristics that help black families to develop, survive, and improve are consistent with Hill's (1972, 1999) analysis of black family strengths. As discussed earlier, these include strong kinship bonds, strong work orientation, strong achievement orientation, adaptability of family roles, and a strong religious orientation. Hill's work stressed the importance of not viewing differences as pathological, and the importance of helping the many different family structures to function as healthily as possible. He warned against 'prejudging [a family's] adequacy on the basis of moral judgments' (Hill, 1999: 22). This is not to deny that black families face real problems, but it is to build recognition of cultures of strength and resistance to racism into the mainstream of social science and social work theories and models. In order to adopt a black perspective when working with black families, social workers need to recognize the strengths in black family systems rooted in 'value orientations different from their own'. Lau proposes that:

> British therapists working with ethnic minority families may be handicapped by a number of factors. They will not possess the same world view as their client families; they will not be aware of how normality and pathology are culturally defined; how the prevailing belief system organizes the perception and behaviour of the group, what is idiosyncratic, and would be accepted by the group as being deviant and what is culturally sanctioned behaviour. They will not be familiar with culturally prescribed rules for sex roles and family roles, and how they are different from rules deriving from Western European cultural context.
>
> (Lau, 2002: 100)

A similar analysis holds true of social work with black families. In addition to understanding the cultural dimension, social workers need to recognize the racism which affects the lives of black people (Sue, 2006). Ahmed notes that:

> The argument is not against better cultural understanding but against an overreliance on cultural explanations, which distract attention both from significant emotional factors, as well as structural factors, such as class and race. The important point is that for Asian clients, the centrality of racism needs to be more explicitly acknowledged in the assessment process, and cultural explanations need to be considered in the context of racism.
>
> (Ahmed, 1981: 65)

Social workers must have an understanding of black kinship ties and family patterns. For instance, as was emphasized earlier, kinship bonds are more extensive in black families than in a white nuclear family.

Many US studies have recognized the important role of the grandmother in the black family (for example, Hill, 1972, 1999; Hale, 1982). Hale, for instance, observed that black grandmothers were more likely to care for their grandchildren and other nonrelated children for extended periods of time, such as foster care and informal adoption, than were their white counterparts. In black families 'kinship ties are much more extensive than in English nuclear family, e.g. a distant cousin is counted as part of the family. This attitude has links in African and Asian history' (Gambe *et al.*, 1992: 34).

The practice of kinship placements is building a strong research base (Farmer and Moyers, 2005). In a study of kinship care, Broad (2001) found that young people and carers highlighted many advantages of such placements over local authority. The advantages included stability; maintaining links with family, siblings and friends; and sustaining and promoting racial and cultural heritage. Social workers need to also be aware that extended family values are an important element in the family assessment. In Britain, immigration controls have made it difficult for 'black family units to be reconstructed in their traditional totality' (Dominelli, 1997: 97). In addition 'poor employment prospects and bad housing also deny black people choices in establishing their preferred family forms. White social workers continue to divide black families by taking disproportionate numbers of black children into care by 'inappropriately intervening in the family process ... [this] has led black people to perceive white social workers as child snatchers' (Dominelli, 1997: 98–9). Social workers need to assess black families in the context of a racist society. They need to be aware that: 'ethnic minority families face many issues ... [which] include personal and institutional racism and the impact of immigration, nationality laws and separated families' (O'Neale, 2000: 1).

However, descriptions of the Asian family in social science literature portray the Asian extended family as being in the process of breaking down due to 'the conflicts and problems Asian men have with their wives, Asian youth have with their parents, Asian girls have with arranged marriages ... [which are] some of the key constructs within which the pathology of the Asian family is embodied' (Parmar, 1981: 24).

Social workers need to identify the strengths of black families, as they can work more efficiently with black clients if they begin from their clients' points of strengths. Graham (2007: 82) notes that empowerment models in social work are closely associated with 'strengths-based approaches ... a strengths perspective serves as the basis for empowerment because this form of practice looks at strengths as the starting point for working in collaboration with clients'.

Acculturation

Social workers need to be aware that acculturation levels (see Chapter 5 for discussion of acculturation) vary not only within cultural groups but also within families (i.e., intergenerational). Different levels of acculturation within families can result in 'disagreement and conflict about family values and parenting behaviours (Zuniga, 1992)' (Bornstein, 1995: 199). Culturally competent social work practice with minority groups should include an assessment of the individual client's acculturation level, as well as an assessment of the family's cultural values, including those of siblings and parents.

Garcia Coll *et al.* (1995: 201) note that 'parents determine, to some extent, familiar ethnic minority aspects of parenting (e.g. disciplinary practices, educational expectations) they uphold and those they relinquish in favor of the dominant culture parental values, attitudes, and practices'.

Racial socialization

Social workers need to understand that racial socialization – particularly how to cope with discrimination, racism, and prejudice – is relevant to understanding the socialization practices of black families. Social workers need to be aware that the socialization of children in black families occurs within the environment of real or potential racial discrimination and prejudice. Thus, according to McAdoo (2002: 59):

> The tasks Black parents share with all parents – providing for and raising children – not only are performed within the mundane extreme environmental stress of racism but include the responsibility of raising physically and emotionally healthy children who are Black in a society in which being Black has negative connotations. This is racial socialization.

In black families, parents often see their primary teaching role as enabling their children to cope with racism (Peters, 1985; Hill, 1999). Peters (1985) found that the black parents 'recognized that being Black brought a different dimension to the way they were raising their children' (Peters, 1985: 171).

Indeed, 'children and adolescents who are socialized about race and ethnicity are further along in identity development than children who are not ... and they demonstrate more positive mental health outcomes and competencies' (Rodriguez *et al.*, 2003: 302).

Social workers must not:

> Ignore the impact that racism and discrimination have on the lives of black people [in Britain] ... today. Both affect a black person from birth until death and have an impact on every aspect of family life, from child-rearing practices, courtship, and marriage, to male-female roles, self-esteem, and cultural and racial identification.
>
> (Boyd-Franklin, 2003: 10)

Barn (2006: 6) argues that 'cultural competence and an understanding of the pernicious effects of institutional and individual racism are pre-requisites for beginning to meet the needs of minority ethnic children and families'. It is crucial for social workers to understand family dynamics, intergenerational struggles, and how the black reality relates to the family's capacity to play its different roles (Devore and Schlesinger, 1981, 1998; McAdoo, 1999).

5 Black identity development

Introduction

For decades, the topic of black identity has been of genuine concern to psychologists and social workers. Low self-esteem, self-hatred, and a negative racial identity have been the characteristics traditionally attributed to black children and adults.

A review of the psychological literature shows that there are different perspectives on the identity development question, which have produced contradictory conclusions.

One body of research which dominated the psychological literature from the early 1940s through to the 1950s is the black self-hatred thesis. Another body of research – developed in the US – focuses on models of psychological nigrescence (a French word that means the 'process of the psychology of becoming black'). A third body of research – developed by African-American researchers – proposes that black personality is in fact Afro-centrically based (Nobles, 1976, 1980, 1986; Williams, 1981; Akbar, 1981a), with an 'African self-consciousness' (Baldwin, 1981) serving as the core for the personality system. He provides clear articulation of the African-American personality in his theory of 'African self-consciousness' (see Baldwin, 1985).

Other approaches to the study of black identity development include ethnic identity formation theory and acculturation theory. The first approach has a more developmental focus, in that it looks at individual change and was originally based on ego identity formation theories. Models of psychological nigrescence are examples of identity development models. The second approach is concerned with the extent to which ethnic identity is maintained when an ethnic minority group is in continuous contact with the dominant group.

This chapter focuses on the black self-hatred thesis, models of racial and ethnic identity development, and acculturation theory. Implications for social work practice are explored.

Some definitions: the terms self-esteem and self-concept have often been used interchangeably. However, self-esteem (or self-worth) has been shown to be one component of self-concept (see, for example, Rosenberg, 1979). According to Mussen *et al.* (1984): 'Self-esteem is based on evaluations and judgements about one's perceived characteristics; self-concept does not imply positive or negative feelings about the self' (1984: 318). On the other hand, the self-concept is 'a set of ideas about oneself that is descriptive rather than judgmental' (Mussen *et al.*, 1984: 356). For example, the fact that black children are aware that they are black is part of the self-concept, but their evaluation of their racial characteristics is part of their self-esteem. Some authors define identity as a component of an individual's overall self-concept. This involves the adoption of certain personal attitudes, feelings, characteristics, and behaviours (personal identity) and the identification with a larger group of people who share those characteristics (reference group orientation).

Black identity has been discussed extensively in the social science literature using various terms and measures. According to Looney, 'Black identity deals specifically with an individual's awareness, values, attitudes, and beliefs about being Black' (1988: 41). It can also be viewed as 'an active developmental process which is exposed to various influences within and without, and [which] can be selective and/or adaptive' (Maxime, 1986: 101). We will use these definitions as our 'operating definition' in our discussion of black identity development.

Overview of black self-hatred research

We shall begin by discussing the group of theories that have been put forward to explain the identity development of blacks, and which have in some way invoked the concept of self-hate and low self-esteem. In fact, Tajfel unequivocally states that:

> There is a good deal of evidence that members of groups which have found themselves for centuries at the bottom of the social pyramid sometimes display the phenomenon of 'self-hate' or 'self-depreciation'. It was one of the merits of the studies on in-group devaluation in children to have provided an accumulation of clear and explicit data on the subject.
>
> (Tajfel, 1982: 12)

One of the most fundamental aspects of identity is the individual's identification with, and preference for, his/her ethnic group. In mainstream psychological literature, a substantial amount of work was produced on black identity. However, most of this work tended to focus on emotional disorder and social pathology among blacks, and there is little research on the topic of psychological health among black people.

Most writers have assumed that, because one's group is an important part of one's self, contempt for one's group by white people (majority) must result in lower self-esteem, and that rejection or hatred of one's group must necessarily reflect rejection of oneself. 'Proshansky and Newton (1968) suggest that the Negro child learns to associate "Negro" with "dirty", "bad", and "ugly", while the white child learns to associate "white" with "clean", "nice" and "good". For the Negro child, these judgements operate to establish his own racial group as inferior to white people' (Nobles, 1973: 18–19). Erikson (1964), too, spoke of ethnic self-doubt and a pathological denial of one's roots as being seminal to Negro identity. He could not conceive that, for some individuals, their colour may actually be a source of pride. In an article, 'Memorandum on identity and Negro youth', he states: 'A lack of familiarity with the problem of Negro youth and with the actions by which Negro youth hopes to solve these problems is a marked deficiency in my life and work which cannot be accounted for by theoretical speculation' (1964: 41).

The mainstream view of black identity has a number of variants. The basic model is that living in a racist white society, where blacks are viewed and treated as inferior and where they are in poverty in a powerless community, leads blacks early in life to internalize negative beliefs and negative feelings about themselves and other blacks. Consequently, the underlying assumption is that exposure to racism and oppression has damaged the black person's psychological make-up, and most probably is reflected in their conceptions of self. The two types of studies in this area were those based on intensive clinical material (Kardiner and Ovessey, 1951) and those based on empirical studies with young children, mostly around their choices and reactions to black and white dolls. These latter studies were particularly influential in promoting the view that black identity implied self-hatred.

Explanations of exactly how the internalization occurs and its precise impacts vary with the theoretical orientation of the writer (see Kardiner and Ovessey, 1951; Pettigrew, 1964; Thomas and Sillen, 1972). The most influential example of the psychological approach has been Kardiner and Ovessey's (1951) *Mark of Oppression* (as mentioned in Chapter 7). They were Freudian psychiatrists, whose central idea was that a group of people who live under the same institutional and environmental conditions will have similar mental and emotional processes, or a 'basic personality' in common. Since American blacks live under similar caste and social class barriers, they should possess a basic personality that differs from that of American whites. In their study, Kardiner and Ovessey (1951) concluded that blacks did have a 'basic personality' that was different and more damaged from that of white Americans. They argued that black personality was centrally organized around adapting to social discrimination (racism). Racist behaviour by whites reveals an unpleasant image of the self to the black individual, who internalizes it and feels worthless, unlovable, and unsuccessful. In essence, he/she feels low self-esteem that eventually is elaborated into self-hatred and idealization of whites. In addition, the frustrations of racist behaviour arouse aggression, which cannot be expressed because of the caste situation, so it must be controlled and contained. Kardiner and Ovessey (1951) argued that this repressed aggression usually led to low self-esteem, depression, and passivity. Grier and Cobbs (1968) used a number of elements of this approach in their discussion of black psychology in the book *Black Rage*. They developed a model of black psychological health that they called the 'Black Norm'. The black norm is a body of personality traits that all American blacks share. 'It also encompasses adaptive devices developed in response to a peculiar environment', which are seen as 'normal devices for making it in America' for blacks (Grier and Cobbs, 1968: 178). The authors contend that the black norm consists of cultural paranoia. They say little about variation by age, class, gender, or region in these characteristics, nor do they provide any non-clinical empirical evidence for them. These psychological models have had substantial theoretical and empirical support (see McCarthy and Yancey, 1971; Taylor, 1976, for reviews). However, more recently a number of authors have challenged these models and approaches. Social scientists have questioned the model's assumptions, noting that, given the social and cultural diversity of the black community, postulating one reaction pattern to racism or one set of personality traits seems unreasonable. Other observers have noted that the black family, institutions, and community can serve as mediators of the negative messages from white society (see Barnes, 1981) and as sources for alternative frames of reference and significant others for black children and adults (see Taylor, 1976). In addition, black identity need not be negative, or may have only an insignificant effect on the psychological functioning or behaviour of the black individual (see Cross, 1980).

Beginning with the early works of Kenneth and Mamie Clark (1939, 1940, 1947, 1950), many studies have attempted to understand the development of racial awareness, preference, identity, and attitudes. Since the work of Kenneth and Mamie Clark is the most widely cited source in the racial identity literature, I shall begin with a discussion of their findings. These studies employed line drawings and photographs of black and white children to assess racial identity in black pre-school children. Subsequently, the Clarks expanded the set of stimulus materials by using dolls and colouring tests (Clark, 1947; Clark, 1965). Most of the research on racial identity has used dolls as stimulus materials. The Clarks introduced the assessment of 'racial preference' into the doll study. Prior to 1947, subjects were required only to identify racial differences and to indicate which stimulus was similar to themselves. The most controversial finding came with the assessment of racial preference. The Clarks (1947) presented 3 to 7-year-old black children with dolls which had identical physiognomies, and differed only with respect to skin and hair colour. The Clarks found that by the age of three, the black children could correctly select the doll that looked 'like a white child' and the one that looked 'like a colored child'. However, when the children were asked 'Give me the nice doll' half chose the white doll. Also, a third of the black children chose the white doll in response to the question 'Give me the doll that looks like you', and half of the black children chose the black doll when asked 'Give me the doll that looks bad'.

This study stimulated a wide body of research (for example, Adelson, 1953; Goodman, 1952; Stevenson and Stewart, 1958). Stevenson and Stewart, for instance, tested 220 children aged 3 to 9 years, of whom 95 were black and 125 were white. This study used the same methodology as the Clarks' research. There were differences between age groups in the black children's choices of the white and brown dolls. Children aged 5–6 years showed the greatest tendency towards white choices for preferred playmates, whereas 59 per cent of the 3-year-olds, and over 60 per cent of the 7-year-olds, made choices favouring the brown doll. Stevenson and Stewart concluded that their findings indicated a higher frequency of negative attitudes towards self among black children. After reviewing the literature, Brand *et al.* state that 'the most consistent finding in this ethnic research is preference by both white and black children for white experimental stimuli' (1974: 883). Black children's preference for the white stimulus has been described as 'white preference behaviour' (Banks, 1976) and 'race dissonance' (Spencer, 1982). In a more recent review of the literature, Tyson (1985) quotes studies that have found a white stimulus preference in other countries, e.g. Gregor and McPherson (1966) in South Africa, Vaughan (1964) in New Zealand, and Milner (1975) and Davey and Mullin (1980) in Britain.

To elaborate on a study carried out in Britain, Milner (1975) studied 100 West Indians, 100 Indians and Pakistanis, and 100 white English children aged between 5 and 8, attending multiracial infant and junior schools in Brixton and Southall in London. Milner used adaptations of the classic doll and picture techniques developed by Clark and Clark (1940) and Morland (1958). The findings were quite clear: West Indian and Asian children in Britain showed a preference for the white majority group and a tendency to devalue their own group.

The Clarks' findings played a major role in the testimony of social scientists in the historic case of *Brown v. Board of Education*, which led to school desegregation (Stephan, 1978). The testimony of Clark and other social scientists suggested that school segregation reinforced black children's feelings of inferiority, which caused low self-esteem. The white preference behaviour observed in these studies was interpreted as evidence of self-rejection and low self-esteem in black children, as they internalize white people's negative view of their race. This view was maintained until the mid-1960s.

Since the late 1960s several studies have contradicted the above studies, showing many black children making more black preference choices than white preference choices (Clark, 1982; Farrell and Olson, 1983; Jordan, 1981; Porter and Washington, 1979) (see summary in Davey, 1987). These studies have shown that black children exhibit positive self-concept and moderate-to-strong black preferences on most of the measures used, i.e. dolls, pictures, direct preference questions, etc. It is argued that black children's personal self-esteem is independent of or compartmentalized from their racial self-esteem (Jordan, 1981).

Banks (1976) asserts that 20 per cent of the twenty-one studies that he considered demonstrated black preference, 10 per cent demonstrated white preference, and 70 per cent showed no preference. In another review of sixteen studies, Aboud and Skerry (1984) found 27 per cent reported black own-group preference, 16 per cent demonstrated white preference, and 57 per cent showed no consensus on preference.

This pro-black trend in the racial preference literature is explained as the social psychological consequences of the 1960s 'black consciousness movement' (e.g. Davey, 1987; Milner, 1983; Hraba and Grant, 1970).

Thus, the pattern of identification and preference among black children is not as unequivocal as was once assumed. A number of arguments have been put forward to explain this discrepancy. Some researchers have criticized the methodology. For example, studies involving preference for photographs or line drawings were criticized because the relative attractiveness of black and white picture stimuli has not always been adequately controlled (Wilkinson, 1974, 1980). Similar criticisms have been levelled against doll selection studies (Baldwin, 1979; Sattler, 1973; Wilkinson, 1974). Brand *et al.* concluded:

> With the range of methodology, control and populations explored in childhood ethnic research, a holistic compilation of results is impossible. Under present empirical and theoretical gaps, it is moot whether studies reflect minority preferences for white stimuli or mirror partial subject responses within biased designs.
>
> (Brand *et al.*, 1974: 883)

In addition to the methodological difficulties of white preference studies, some authors have questioned the basic assumptions on which this type of research is based. Most researchers have found that whites tend to prefer white stimuli and have held to the implicit assumption that such preference behaviour is normal. However Nobles (1973) raised serious questions about the validity of such an assumption, and contends that the behaviour of whites should not be the norm against which other groups are judged.

Other authors have argued that black children's failure to identify with the black doll was due to the particular economic and social contexts within which the children find themselves, and not a general deficit in self-esteem (Fine and Bowers, 1984). Cross (1985) indicated that racially symbolic assessments and direct assessments tap different dimensions of children's self-concept: reference-group orientation and personal identity, respectively (see Cross, 1985, for detailed review).

Another difficulty that has arisen with respect to racial preference research has been the failure of researchers, and interpreters of research, to recognize the developmental constraints of white preference behaviour (Spencer, 1988). Spencer (1984) carried out a study of 130 black children, aged between 4 and 6.5 years old, to assess the relationships between self-concept, race awareness, and racial attitudes (including racial preferences). She used racial picture cards and paper-doll cutouts, a self-concept values test, and a vocabulary measure. Spencer found that 80 per cent of the children obtained positive self-concept scores, and at the same time showed an anti-black/white preference in their racial attitudes. Spencer concluded that black pre-schoolers are able to effectively compartmentalize their self-concept from their racial attitudes. Banks (1984) found that black children from predominantly white communities and schools tended to have positive self-concepts and to be anti-black/pro-white in their racial attitudes and preferences. He referred to this phenomenon as a 'biracial' orientation.

In an inquiry into the assumptions underlying self-esteem and minority status, Rosenberg (1979) suggests that most theoretical formulations assuming a relationship between the two rest largely on two concepts: reflected appraisals and social comparisons. The principle of reflected appraisals assumes that self-concept is largely built up by adopting the attitudes of others towards the self, and it follows therefore that, if others look down on the minority group, it will come to see itself more or less as they do. While accepting that principle, Rosenberg (1979) points out that the conversion of society's attitude towards one's group, into the individual's attitude towards the self, is possible only if certain assumptions are made. The first is that the individual knows how the majority feels about his/her group (the assumption of awareness); the second is that he/she accepts the societal view of the group (the assumption of agreement); the third is that he/she accepts these views as being applicable to him/herself (the assumption of personal relevance); and fourth is that he/she is critically concerned with majority attitudes (the assumption of significance). Rosenberg presents empirical evidence to show that these conditions must be met if the principle of reflected appraisals is to hold. Rosenberg believes that black children compare themselves with other blacks, not with whites, and that they do so on the basis of the structure of the environment in which they live.

The self-hatred thesis is accurate in acknowledging the fact that white society in America and Britain provides no positive images through which blacks could see themselves reflected in a positive way. However, it is inaccurate in assuming that black people look to whites as their only source of validation and emulation. This perspective ignores the necessity for black people to use themselves and their culture (and their history) as primary referents. Baldwin states that the black self-hatred research proposes that:

> Black people, especially children, acquire their self-conception from their interaction with the Euro-American community rather than from the African American community ... the illogical basis of such an assertion has been effectively demonstrated by many black social scientists and some white social scientists as well (Baldwin, 1979; Nobles, 1973; Porter & Washington, 1979).
>
> (Baldwin, 1991: 152)

Whatever the explanation, the conclusions of research showing that children may show preferences for the white stimuli cannot be ignored. Some contemporary studies show that many black children continue to make white preference or anti-black racial evaluations (Banks, 1984; Clark, 1982; McAdoo, 1985; Gopaul-McNicol, 1988; Powell-Hopson, 1985; Semaj, 1980; Spencer, 1984). For example, in a study of racial identification and racial preference of black pre-school children in New York and Trinidad, Gopaul-McNicol (1988) found that the results of their study were very similar to Clark and Clark's (1947) findings in that the majority of the black children showed a preference for the white doll, and identified with the white doll. The study indicates that there has been little change in the racial attitudes of black pre-school children over the past forty years (Gopaul-McNicol, 1988). In a recent study of ethnic/racial attitudes and self-identification of black Jamaican and white New England Children, Cramer and Anderson (2003: 395) found that 'overall [all the] children showed white favoritism'.

In Britain, Davey and Norburn (1980) found that only a third of their 7-year-old West Indian sample in London and Yorkshire, and two-thirds of their 10-year-old sample, chose the photograph of the child in their own racial group as the one 'they would most like to be'. The proportion of Asian and West Indian children who made 'own group choices' at both age levels was very similar. White children of the same age still showed an overwhelming level of 'own group preference'. In a study of ethnic preferences and perceptions among Asian and white British middle school children, Boulton and Smith (1992: 55) found that although 'Asian and White children selected an own-race photograph as being most like them, ... only about a half [of Asian children] selected the own-race photograph as the one they would most like to be'. Banks (2003: 158) observes that 'when black children "judge" or evaluate their own group attributes using the racist notions of others, they enter a process of internalizing racism and, in effect devalue themselves in devaluing their racial group'.

Although most black people in Britain 'possess the survival skills necessary for the development of a positive racial identity ... [there are those] who experience difficulty in maintaining a positive sense of racial identity' (Maxime, 1986: 101). Thus, the need for greater participation by parents, social workers, and educators in the promotion of racial pride and self-acceptance in black children is still urgent today (Maxime, 1997).

Models of black identity development

From the mainstream psychological research literature on black identity examined in the above section, I want to move the focus to a perspective that has largely been ignored by traditional Eurocentric psychology

– research on the psychology of nigrescence. The literature on black self-hatred suggests the operation of a basic Eurocentric position in psychology and social science, at least where the issues of race and racial differences are concerned (Baldwin, 1976; Clark (X), 1972). The preoccupation with self-hatred has kept researchers from discovering black strengths. In 1971 Cedrick Clark declared that 'the language of contemporary psychology, particularly dealing with black Americans, is basically monodic: phenomena are described in terms of entities and characteristics which a person processes instead of the processes in which he/she is engaged' (Clark, 1971: 33).

The study of nigrescence developed in the late 1960s as black American psychologists tried to outline the identity transformation that accompanied an individual's participation in the Black power phase (1968–75) of the Black Social Movement. Nigrescence models tend to have four or five stages – and the common point of departure is not the change process per se but an analysis of the identity to be changed. These models are useful as they enable us to understand the problems of black identity confusion and to examine, at a detailed level, what happens to a person during identity change. However, as Cross (1980) points out, it is important to remember that nigrescence models 'speak to the phenomenon of identity metamorphosis within the context of a social movement and not the evolution of identity from childhood through adult life' (Cross, 1980: 97).

The traditional psychological literature on black identity tended to have children as subjects (for example, the doll studies), whereas the nigrescence approach studies black identity in adolescents and adults. Parham considers that:

> The process of psychological Nigrescence (the development of Black racial identity attitudes) is a lifelong process, which begins with the late-adolescence/early-adulthood period in an individual's life .... Manifestations of Black identity at earlier stages of a youngster's life (childhood) may be a reflection of externalized parental attitudes or societal stereotypes that a youngster has incorporated (Spencer, 1982) rather than a crystallized personal identity.
>
> (Parham, 1989: 194–5)

Several models of black identity development and transformation were introduced in the early 1970s. Each model hypothesized that identity development was characterized by movement across a series of sequential stages, and that changes were influenced by an individual's reaction to social and environmental pressures and circumstances (Cross, 1971,

1978; Jackson, 1975; Thomas and Thomas, 1971; Williams, 1975). For example, Thomas described a five-step process that he proposed as a necessary condition for black people to destroy 'Negromachy'. This term is defined by Thomas as domination by a confusion of self-worth, and dependence on white society for definition of self:

> Inherent in this concept of approval is the need to be accepted as something other than what one is. Gratification is based upon denial of self and a rejection of group goals and activities. The driving force behind this need requires Afro-Americans to seek approval from whites in all activities, to use white expectations as the yard stick for determining what is good, desirable or necessary.
>
> (Thomas and Thomas, 1971: 104)

Jackson (1975) put forward a Black Identity Development Theory (BID) that describes the process by which a black person develops a positive racial identity.

Perhaps the best known and most widely researched model of black identity development is Cross's (1971, 1978, 1980) model of the conversion from 'Negro' to 'black'. Cross suggests that the development of a black person's racial identity is often characterized by his/her movement through a five-stage process, the transformation from pre-encounter to internalization-commitment. The five stages are:

1   Pre-encounter. In the first stage the person is likely to view the world from a white frame of reference (Eurocentric). The black person accepts a 'white' view of self, other blacks, and the world. The person has accepted a deracinated frame of reference and because his or her reference point is usually a white normative standard, he or she develops attitudes that are very pro-white and anti-black. The person will also deny that racism exists. Cross stresses that this stage 'is in evidence across social class' (Cross *et al.*, 1991: 323).
    Cross *et al.* state that:

> At the core of the Stage 1 description is an aggressive assimilation-integration agenda, an agenda linked not only to the search for a secure place in the socio-economic mainstream, but motivated as well by a desperate attempt to escape from the implications of being a 'Negro'. In this light, the Stage 1 Negro is depicted as a deracinated person who views being black as an obstacle, problem or stigma and seldom a symbol of culture, tradition or struggle. The Negro is thus preoccupied with the thoughts of how to overcome

his stigma, or how he can assist whites in discovering that he is 'just another human being' who wants to assimilate.

(Cross *et al.*, 1991: 322–3)

2   Encounter. In the second stage some shocking personal or social event makes the person receptive to new views of being black and of the world. The person's Eurocentric thinking is upset by an encounter with racial prejudice and precipitates an intense search for black identity. The encounter stage involves two steps: first, experiencing and personalizing the event – the person realizes that his/her old frame of reference is inappropriate, and he/she begins to explore aspects of a new identity; the second part is portrayed by Cross *et al.* 'as a testing phase during which the individual [first] cautiously tries to validate his/her new perceptions' (Cross *et al.*, 1991: 324), then definitively decides to develop a black identity.

Consequently, when the person absorbs enough information and receives enough social support to conclude that: (1) the old identity seems inappropriate and (2) the proposed new identity is highly attractive, the person starts an obsessive and extremely motivated search for black identity. At the end of the second stage the person is not depicted as having obtained the new identity, but as having made the decision to start the journey towards the new identity. The person feels less internally secure and seeks authentication through external validation.

3   Immersion-Emersion. 'This stage encompasses the most sensational aspects of black identity development' (Cross, 1971). This is the period of transition in which the person struggles to destroy all vestiges of the 'old' perspective. This occurs simultaneously with an intense concern to clarify the personal implications of the new-found black identity (Cross, 1978). An emotional period ensues where the person glorifies anything black and attempts to purge him or herself of their former worldview and old behaviour. The old self is regarded in pejorative terms, but the person is unfamiliar with the new self, for that is what he/she hopes to become; 'thus the person is forced to erect simplistic, glorified, highly romantic and speculative images of what he or she assumes the new self will be like' (Cross *et al.*, 1991: 325). The person begins to immerse him/herself into total blackness. He/she attaches himself/herself to black culture and at the same time withdraws from interactions with white people. The person tends to denigrate white people and white culture, thus exhibiting anti-white attitudes. Cross *et al.* state: 'Since the new black identity is something yet to be achieved, the Stage 3 person

is generally anxious about how to demonstrate to others that he/she is becoming the right kind of black person' (Cross *et al.*, 1991: 325). Hence, the demonstration of one's blackness is prominent – for example, black clothes and hairstyles, linguistic style, attending all black functions, reading black literature. The person does not feel secure about his/her blackness. He/she can be vicious in attacks on aspects of the old self that appear in others or his/herself, and he/she may even appear bizarre in his/her affirmation of the new self. The potential personal chaos of this stage is generally tempered by the social support a person gains through group activities. The groups joined during this period are 'counterculture institutions', which have rituals, obligations, and reward systems that nurture and reward the developing identity, while inhibiting the efficacy of the 'old identity'. Although the initial part of Stage 3 involves total immersion and personal withdrawal into blackness, the latter part of this stage represents emergence from the reactionary, 'either-or' and racist aspects of the immersion experience. The person's emotions begin to level off, and psychological defensiveness is replaced by affective and cognitive openness. This allows the person to be more critical in his/her analysis of what it means to be black. The strengths, weaknesses, and oversimplifications of blackness can now be sorted out as the person's degree of ego-involvement diminishes and his/her sense of perspective expands. The person begins to feel in greater control of himself/herself and the most difficult period of nigrescence comes to an end.

4   Internalization. In this stage, the person focuses on things other than himself/herself and his/her ethnic or racial group. He/she achieves an inner security and self-confidence with his/her blackness. He/she feels more relaxed, more at ease with self. The person's thinking reflects a shift from how friends see him/her (Am I black enough?) towards confidence in personal standards of blackness. The person also exhibits a psychological openness and a decline in strong anti-white feelings. The person still uses 'blacks as a primary reference group, [but] moves towards a pluralistic and nonracist perspective' (Cross, 1991: 326). Thus: 'As internalization and incorporation increase, attitudes toward White people become less hostile, or at least realistically contained, and pro-Black attitudes become more expansive, open and less defensive' (Cross, 1971: 24).

This stage, and the fifth stage of internalization-commitment, are characterized by positive self-esteem, ideological flexibility, and openness about one's blackness. In the fifth stage the person finds activities and commitments to express his/her new identity. Cross (1985) contends that:

> Implicit in the distinction between 'internalization' and 'internalization-commitment' is the proposition that in order for Black identity change to have 'lasting political significance', the 'self' (me or 'I') must become or continue to be involved in the resolution of problems shared by the 'group' (we).
>
> (Cross, 1985: 86)

There is an extensive empirical literature that confirms Cross's model of black identity development (see Cross, 1971; Hall *et al.*, 1972; Marks *et al.*, 2004; Milliones, 1973; Williams, 1975; Wijeyesinghe and Jackson, 2001). One very good example of Cross's model can be seen in the autobiography of Malcolm X (1965). According to Cross (1985) the evolution from the pre-encounter to the internalization stage reflects a movement from psychological dysfunction to psychological health (Vandiver, 2001).Cross sees the person in stage five – internalization-commitment – as the 'ideal'; that is, a psychologically healthy black person. They have made their new pro-black identity and values their own. They have a 'calm, secure demeanor' characterized by 'ideological flexibility, psychological openness and self-confidence about one's blackness' (Cross, 1980: 86). Blacks are a primary reference group, but the person has lost his/her prejudices about race, sex, age, and social class. He/she also struggles to translate his/her values into behaviour that will benefit the black community. According to Cross *et al.*:

> For the person who has reached Stage 4 and beyond, the internalized black identity tends to perform three dynamic functions: to defend and protect a person from psychological insults, and where possible to warn of impending psychological attacks that stem from having to live in a racist society; to provide social anchorage and meaning to one's existence by establishing black people as a primary reference group; to serve as a point of departure for gaining awareness about, and completing transactions with, the broader world of which blackness is but a part.
>
> (Cross *et al.*, 1991: 328)

In summary, the research suggests that:

1   Many blacks have a predominantly positive racial identity, with perhaps a minority having a negative identity.

2 Black identity has links to behaviour.
3 Black identity can have links to other attitudes and personality characteristics.

However, the issue of whether an individual's type (positive, negative) of black identity is linked to their level of personal self-esteem seems unresolved. While Cross (1985) and Clark (1982) find no evidence for such a link, Gibbs (1974) and Parham and Helms (1985) do find empirical evidence.

More recently, Cross (1995, *et al.* 1998, 2001) has proposed revisions in the conceptualizations of nigrescence. His recent descriptions of the stages depict a more diverse set of attitudes and behaviours associated with the different stages than he originally described. Cross (*et al.* 1998, 2002) has recognized that the original definitions of the Pre-encounter and internalization stages may have been limited by their focus on single dimensions in each stage. In the case of the pre-encounter stage, he now posits a continuum of racial attitudes that extend from low salience, to race neutral, to anti-black. Thus, a person with pre-encounter attitudes may acknowledge his or her blackness while believing that it has little importance or meaning in their life (low salience). He/she value things 'other than their blackness, such as their religion, their lifestyle, their social status, or their profession' (Cross 1995: 98); or he or she may express strong anti-black sentiments as a way of denigrating the culture and distancing themselves from other African Americans who are perceived to be 'too black' for their personal comfort. Thus, not all black people place race and black culture at the center of their identity (Cross and Fhagen-Smith, 1996). For some, social identity or reference group orientation may be grounded in religious ideas, or the fact that they are gay or lesbian, whereas for others, race, ethnicity, and black culture are at the core of their existence (Cross, 1995). According to Cross (1998) *low salience* identities (LS) refer to black social identities or reference-group orientations that accord only minor significance to race and African American culture in determining what is, and is not, important in one's everyday life; *high salience* identities (HS) characterize black social identities for which race and African culture are of central significance. Adolescence is the period during which a broad range of LS and HS social identities come to fruition. It is also the point at which LS identities may be changed by a Nigrescence conversion (Cross, 1995, *et al.* 1998).

With regard to the internalization stage, Cross (1995, 2001) now takes the position that an individual's resolution of internalized attitudes will also vary, for example, from a monocultural focus (nationalistic) to one that is more multicultural in orientation. In either case, as with the pre-encounter stage, it is important to remember that the nigrescence process does not evolve into a single ideological stance. Rather, there is a multitude of ways in which one's cultural pride and internalized identity may be expressed.

The five stages of black identity development, however, remain the same. Cross also notes that the immersion-emersion stage can result in regression, fixation or stagnation, instead of continued identity development. Regression refers to those people 'whose overall experience is negative and thus non-reinforcing of growth toward the new identity [and therefore] may become disappointed and choose to reject Blackness' (Cross, 1991: 208). Some people can become fixated at this stage due to extreme and negative encounters with white racists. Thus: 'Individuals who experience painful perceptions and confrontations will be overwhelmed with hate for white people and fixated at stage 3' (Cross, 1991: 208). Finally, dropping out of any involvement with black issues is another response to the immersion-emersion stage. Some people might drop out because they wish to 'move on to what they perceive as more important issues in life' (Cross, 1991: 209). These people tend to label their experience as their 'ethnicity phase'. Cross has noted that this often occurs with African American college students.

There are multiple ways in which black identity operates or functions in one's daily life. The five key identity operations for conducting a functional analysis of black identity include: buffering; bonding; bridging; code-switching, and individualism (Clark, Swim and Cross, 1995; Cross, 1991; Cross, Parham and Helms, 1995). The buffering function refers to those ideas, attitudes, feelings, and behaviors that accord psychological protection and self-defence against everyday encounters with racism. The person either anticipates what might be avoided, or employs a buffer to blunt the sting and pain arising from an unavoidable or unsuspecting racist encounter. HS African Americans tend to recognize potential racist encounters in everyday American life, and consider the development and constant refinement of the buffering mechanism to be crucial to their psychological integrity. Conversely, LS African Americans stress a colour-blind perspective and tend to see less racism in everyday American life.

The bonding function addresses the degree to which the person derives meaning and support from an affiliation with or attachment to black people and black culture. HS African Americans place importance to their attachment to black people and black culture. LS African Americans tend to exhibit less attachment and affiliation to black culture.

The bridging function refers to those competencies, attitudes, and behaviors that make it possible for a black person to immerse himself or herself in another group's experience, absent of any need to suppress one's sense of blackness. The person moves back and forth between black culture and the ways of knowing, acting, thinking, and feeling that constitute a non-black worldview. During these bridging transactions, no demands are made on either party to deny his or her cultural frame of reference.

Some HS African Americans who embrace a black nationalist or Afrocentric perspective may not place much value in bridging, preferring to concentrate their time and energy on black (in-group) tasks and problems. Some HS African Americans, who are as comfortable by that which makes them American as that which makes them black (biculturality) or who relish sharing experiences with a range of other groups (multiculturality), are more likely to use the bridging function. LS African Americans may have experiences across racial and cultural divides, not out of a sense of cultural or ethnic bridging, but because their colour-blind philosophy makes out-group friendships and experiences possible.

The buffering, bonding, and bridging functions of black identity have been identified by Cross (1991) as well as Cross *et al.*, (1995). More recently, Clark *et al.* (1995) extended the list to include codeswitching and individualism. The codeswitching function allows a person to temporarily accommodate to the norms and regulations of a group, organization, school, or workplace. Finally, individualism is the expression of one's unique personality.

Although Cross's identity development model has been developed with African-American samples in the US, it is argued by various authors (for example, Maxime, 1986; Sue and Sue, 1990; Sue, 2006) that other minority groups share similar processes of development. For instance, Sue (2006: 92) indicates that:

> 'Earlier writers (Berry, 1965; Stonequist, 1937) have observed that minority groups share similar patterns of adjustment to cultural oppression. In the past several decades, [in the USA] Asian Americans, Hispanics, and American Indians have experienced sociopolitical identity transformations so that a 'Third World consciousness' has emerged with a cultural oppression as the common unifying force.
> (Sue, 2006: 92)

If a black person, Baldwin (1985) asserts, is exposed to an environment which is unsupportive, denigrating, oppressive, and even hostile, and affirmation and validation for one's existence is lacking or non-existent, then a negative sense of self is a likely outcome, with the models of nigrescence serving as an appropriate explanation of the resolution process that self will likely experience (also see Helms, 2003). Sue and Sue (1999: 124) point out that 'early models of racial identity development all incorporated the effects of racism and prejudice (oppression) upon the identity transformation of their victims'.

In Britain, Robinson (2000) compared the racial identity attitudes and self-esteem of African Caribbean adolescents in residential care in a city in the West Midlands, and a group of African Caribbean adolescents living with their own families and attending a multi-racial school in the city. Both respondents in residential care and the comparison group primarily endorsed positive racial attitudes. Self-esteem and racial identity attitudes were positively related. Residential care staff found Cross's model extremely useful in therapeutic work with African Caribbean children. Maxime (1986) has used Cross's model in the understanding of identity confusion in black adolescents and adults. However, she points out that 'difficulty in maintaining a positive sense of racial identity does not apply to all black people' (Maxime, 1986: 101).

Parham's lifespan nigrescence model

Perhaps the most important theoretical advance in the field of nigrescence is Parham's application of a lifespan perspective to the study of nigrescence. In Cross's model, nigrescence was regarded as a 'one-time event' in the person's life cycle.

Parham (1989) proposed that identity development may recycle throughout adulthood. Some people may have completed the nigrescence cycle at an early stage in the life cycle – for example, in adolescence or adulthood – but they may find that the challenges unique to a later phase in the life cycle – for example, middle age or late adulthood – may bring about a recycling through some of the stages.

Parham presents a life-cycle nigrescence model based on a modification of the Cross model. Parham is concerned to identify the earliest phase of the life cycle at which a person is capable of experiencing nigrescence. He argues that the 'manifestations of Black identity [during childhood] may be a reflection of externalized parental attitudes or societal stereotypes that a youngster has incorporated (Spencer, 1982) rather than a crystallized personal identity' (Parham, 1989: 95). Accordingly, he proposes that it is during adolescence and early adulthood that a person might first experience nigrescence, and after this first experience, the likelihood of experiencing nigrescence is present for the rest of a person's life. Parham's model assumes that there is a qualitative difference between the nigrescence experience at adolescence or in early adulthood and, say, in middle or late adulthood, because:

> A Black person's frame of reference is potentially influenced by his or her life stage and the developmental tasks associated with that period of life ... [and] within the context of normal development, racial identity is a phenomenon which is subject to continuous change during the life cycle.
>
> (Parham, 1989: 196)

While Cross's model demonstrates how a person's racial identity can change from one stage to another (i.e., pre-encounter to encounter to immersion-emersion to internalization), it has failed to indicate how the different stages of racial identity will be emphasized at different phases of the life cycle. However, Parham's model describes the stages of racial identity at different phases of life (see Parham, 1989, for full discussion).

A person's racial identity development does not have to begin with a pro-white/anti-black viewpoint (pre-encounter stage). For instance, 'if an adolescent is raised in a home environment in which the parents have strong Immersion-Emersion attitudes, then [Parham] ... speculates that [the adolescent's] attitudes are likely to be Immersion-Emersion as well' (Parham, 1989: 213).

Parham proposes three different ways in which a person deals with his/her racial identity as he/she advances through life: stagnation, stage-wise linear progression, and recycling. Stagnation is defined 'as maintaining one type of race-related attitude throughout most of one's lifetime' (Parham, 1989: 211). The stage-wise linear progression refers to the 'movement from one stage to another in a stage-to-stage fashion (i.e., pre-encounter to internalization) over a period of time in one's life' (Parham, 1989: 213). Recycling is defined as:

> The reinitiation into the racial identity struggle and resolution process after having gone through the identity process at an earlier stage in one's life. In essence, a person could theoretically achieve identity resolution by completing one cycle through the nigrescence process (internalization) and, as a result of ... identity confusion, recycle through the stages again.
>
> (Parham, 1989: 213)

It is apparent from the growing body of theoretical activity that racial identity is becoming a major theoretical and empirical model in psychology (Carter, 1995; Helms, 1990; Helms and Piper, 1994; Marks *et al.*, 2004; Sue, 2006).

Ethnic identity development model

Another theoretical approach to the study of black adolescents' identity development is ethnic identity formation theory. Since the 1970s, racial, ethnic or minority identity theories have been introduced to include other visible racial/ethnic groups. Ethnic identity 'a) concerns one's attachment to and sense of belonging to, and identification with one's ethnic group members (e.g., Japanese, Indian) and with one's ethnic culture; b) does not have a theoretical emphasis on oppression/racism; but c) may include the prejudices and cultural pressures that ethnic individuals experience when their ways of life come into conflict with those of the White dominant group' (Sodowsky *et al.*, 1995: 132).

Tajfel (1981) defines ethnic identity as 'that part of an individual's self-concept which derives from his knowledge of his membership of a social group (or groups) together with the value and emotional significance attached to that membership' (1981: 255). Other definitions and interpretations of ethnicity include: self-identification; feelings of belongingness and commitment; and the sense of shared values and attitudes (see Phinney, 1990).

According to Rotheram and Phinney (1987) 'ethnic identity refers to one's sense of belonging to an ethnic group and the part of one's thinking, perceptions, feelings, and behaviour that is due to ethnic group membership' (1987: 13). Phinney (1989) views the process of ethnic identity development as a progression through a series of stages. The model proposed by Phinney (1989) is congruent with Cross's racial identity development discussed above. This congruence is based on the fact that Phinney's model is rooted in the ego identity development literature by sharing the idea that an achieved identity occurs through stages and is the result of a crisis, an awakening, and/or an encounter. This leads to a period of exploration or experimentation, and finally to a commitment or incorporation of one's ethnicity. Apart from focusing mainly on adolescents, Phinney's model differs from the others by reducing the number of stages contained in the model.

Phinney's (1989) model of ethnic identity development in adolescence is therefore made up of three stages. The first stage is known as unexamined ethnic identity (i.e. individuals at this stage are not in the process of exploring ethnicity). This may be accompanied by lack of interest or concern with the subject (diffusion) or by attitudes about one's ethnicity that are derived from others (foreclosure). These attitudes 'may be either positive or negative, depending on one's socialization experiences' (Phinney, 1989: 38). Phinney holds that the diffused and foreclosed statuses from Marcia are similar to each other. With foreclosure, individuals either have accepted the majority culture's values and attitudes, or in the diffuse status, the adolescent may not have been exposed to ethnic identity issues. In both the diffuse and foreclosed states, the adolescent has not examined his or her ethnic identity, and is therefore in Phinney's 'unexamined' first stage. In the second stage, ethnic identity search (moratorium), individuals are involved in exploring and seeking to understand the meaning of ethnicity for themselves. This exploration may be triggered by a significant 'awakening' experience around their ethnicity that often is followed by 'an intense process of immersion in one's own culture through activities such as reading, talking to people, going to ethnic museums, and participating actively in cultural events' (Phinney, 1989: 38). Through this process, Phinney argued, individuals come to a deeper understanding of what their ethnic identity means to them. A third component of Phinney's model emphasizes individual's feelings with respect to their affirmation and belonging towards their ethnic group. Specifically, this component consists of one's feelings of ethnic pride, feeling good about one's background, and being happy with one's group. The final component, ethnic identity achievement, stresses the idea that ethnic identity is dynamic. Phinney developed the Multi-group Ethnic Identity Measure (MEIM) to measure these various universal components of ethnic identity (Phinney, 1992). Phinney and Kohatsu (1997: 420) note that 'For adolescents of color, the successful transition to healthy functioning in adulthood requires the achievement of a secure sense of their ethnic and/or racial identity, in the face of stereotypical images of their group, cultural differences and conflicts, and restricted opportunities ... this process, which is typically neither salient nor important for white adolescents, is of central importance to American [and British] adolescents from non-European backgrounds'.

Critique of stage models

Stage theories of ethnic identity development have been criticized by some researchers as being too linear, and not recognizing the multi-dimensional nature of ethnic identity (e.g. Yeh and Huang, 1996). Many stage theories fail to capture the complexity and uniqueness of the ethnic minority experience. For example, the stage model for minority identity development proposed by Atkinson *et al.* (1983) has received scrutiny and criticism from the psychology field. Jones (1991) argues that this model is too linear; there is no explanation of what factors contribute to or promote progression on to the next stage. This model also does not fully acknowledge the dominant society's role in the continuing cycle of racism in the United States and Britain (Helms, 1986). Furthermore, Jones (1991) argues that the model of ethnic identity development proposed by Atkinson *et al.* (1983) places the blame of racism on the victim – suggesting and encouraging change in the ethnic group – and not on the majority group's attitudes and behaviours. A final criticism of ethnic identity development models is that there are few majority group identity models, thus placing emphasis on minority group differences. Because US and British society includes various cultural groups and influences, theories should emphasize cultural similarities as well as differences. However, the conceptual models that have been proposed in the literature are useful in understanding the experiences of black and minority adolescents in US and Britain (Trimble *et al.*, 2003; Sue and Sue, 2003; Sue, 2006).

Acculturation

Acculturation theory is similar to the models discussed earlier (Cross, 1978; Phinney, 1989) in its emphasis on a conflict model of ethnic identity. Both theories assume there will be an apparent conflict for ethnic minorities because of being part of two different cultural systems – the minority group to which they belong and the majority or dominant group. However, acculturation theorists (e.g. Berry, 1990) argue that 'acculturation may be a more complex and multi-dimensional concept, so that a simple stage model will hardly do justice to the process whereby an individual comes to terms with his or her ethnic identity' (Coleman and Hendry, 1999: 65). Ethnic identity is an aspect of acculturation that is concerned with how individuals feel about or relate to their own ethnic group as part of the larger majority or dominant society. Acculturation theory, then, is concerned with the extent to which ethnic identity is maintained when an ethnic group is in continuous contact with the dominant group (Phinney, 1990).

Phinney (1999: 27) points out that:

> Within multicultural industrialized nations, issues of cultural contact and the resulting identity conflicts are most obvious among immigrants and the children of immigrants, who on a daily basis face exposure to differing cultural expectations. Children of

immigrants are confronted with the task of constructing an identity by selecting or combining elements from their culture of origin and from the new culture in which they are growing up.

The concept of psychology of acculturation was introduced by Graves (1967). It refers to changes in an individual who is a participant in a culture contact situation, being influenced both directly by the external culture, and by the changing culture of which the individual is a member. The main reason for keeping these two levels distinct is that not every individual enters into, or participates and changes, the same way. This literature has been extensively reviewed by Berry (1997), Liebkind (2000) and Ward (1996). Garcia Coll (*et al.* 1995: 199) writes that 'the process of acculturation is important not only for immigrants but also for any individual who for historic, economic, political, linguistic, and/or religious reasons is exposed or expected to adapt to a new cultural environment'.

While acculturation is a neutral term in principle (that is, change may take place in either or both groups), in practice acculturation tends to induce more change in the immigrant group. There are vast individual differences in how people attempt to deal with acculturative change (Berry, 1997). These strategies (termed acculturation strategies) have three aspects: their preferences ('acculturation attitudes'; see Berry *et al.*, 1989); how much change they actually undergo ('behavioural shifts'; see Berry, 1980); and how much of a problem these changes are for them (the phenomenon of 'acculturative stress'; see Berry *et al.*, 1987).

Berry (1990) has suggested that the acculturation strategies of ethnic minority groups can best be described in terms of two independent dimensions: 1) retention of one's cultural traditions, and 2) establishment and maintenance of relationships with the larger society. When these two central dimensions are considered simultaneously, a conceptual framework is generated which posits four acculturation strategies.

Acculturation strategies involve: assimilation, integration, separation and marginalization. If individuals do not wish to maintain their own cultural identity, and seek daily interaction with other cultures, then the Assimilation strategy is defined. In contrast, when non-dominant persons place a value on holding onto their original culture, and at the same time wish to avoid interaction with others, then the Separation alternative is defined. When this mode of acculturation is pursued by the dominant group with respect to the non-dominant group, then the term Separation is appropriate. When there is an interest in both maintaining one's original culture, and in daily interactions with other groups, Integration is the option; here, there is some degree of cultural integrity maintained, while at the same time moving to participate as an integral part of the larger social network. Finally, when there is little possibility or interest in cultural maintenance, and little interest in relations with others, Marginalization is defined. Attitudes towards these four alternatives, and the actual behaviours exhibiting them, together constitute an individual's acculturation strategy. Substantial evidence now exists showing that individuals who pursue the integration strategy have the most positive adaptation, while those who are marginalized by the process of acculturation are least well adapted; assimilation and separation lie in between, one or the other being the more successful depending on the group and their situation (Berry and Sam, 1997; Phinney *et al.*, 1992).

This presentation of attitudinal positions is based on the assumption that immigrants have the freedom to choose how they want to engage in intercultural relations. However, this is not always the case (Berry, 1974). For example, a mutual accommodation is required for Integration to be attained, involving the acceptance by both the dominant and non-dominant group of the right of all groups to live as culturally different peoples within the same society. This strategy requires immigrants to adopt the basic values of the national society, while at the same time the national society must be prepared to adapt national institutions (e.g. education, health, justice, employment) to better meet the needs of all groups now living together in the larger plural society.

Berry's model is more useful than a linear, one-dimensional model. However, a

> major shortcoming of [Berry's] model is that it underplays the significance of the attitudes, values and the zeitgeist of the receiving society. The decision to integrate or not to integrate does not entirely rest on the immigrants and their descendants, but also – perhaps more so – on the reaction of the host society.
>
> (Ghuman, 1999: 35)

Phinney and Devich-Navarro (1997: 26) argue that: 'The attitudes of the larger society toward the ethnic group are clearly an important influence on the extent to which individuals feel bicultural'. The authors note that 'a determining factor in one's cultural identification appears to be the individual's perception of society; to feel bicultural, one must see the larger society as inclusive' (1997: 26).

In addition, 'Both racial identity theory and studies of cultural or ethnic identity suggest that individuals need to explore and become secure in their own cultural background as part of the process of accepting other groups and the larger society' (Phinney and Devich-Navarro, (1997: 28).

There is little empirical evidence about how individuals from ethnic minority groups in Britain think about and handle their relationship with the two cultures in which they live. Very little empirical work using Berry's acculturation model has been conducted in Britain. It helps us to explore the adaptation strategies of minority groups living in Britain (Ghuman, 1999; Robinson, 2003).

In Britain, studies of young Asian people have shown that most young people prefer the integration mode of adaptation (Ghuman, 1997; Hutnik, 1991; Robinson, 2003; Stopes-Roe and Cochrane, 1990). Ghuman (1997) found differences within the Asian group. For instance, Hindu young people were more in favour of taking up English values and ways of life than Muslims. Sikh young people came somewhere in-between Hindus and Muslims as judged by their performance on the scale.

Studies of Asians in Britain (e.g. Anwar, 1978; Robinson, 2003; Shaw, 1988) indicate that first generation Asians employed 'separation' as a mode of working and living in Britain. In his study of Asian adolescents, Ghuman (1999: 69) found that 'the majority of young [Asian] people prefer integration to other modes of adaptation (for example, assimilation, marginalization and separation) [and this] is reinforced by the face-to-face interview data'. Thus, Ghuman found that 'a large majority of young [Asian] people are bi-cultural and bi-lingual: they have retained some aspects of their own culture and at the same time adopted some of the British norms. ... the majority define their personal identity in a "hyphenated way" (for example, Indo-English)'(1999: 69). However, 'this has not changed the fact that they continue to suffer racial abuse both in and out of school and have mixed feelings about whether they belong [in Britain]'(Ghuman, 2003: 130).

In a recent study undertaken as part of the International Comparative Study of Ethnocultural Youth, Robinson (2003) found that the acculturation attitude most favoured by Indian, Pakistani and African Caribbean adolescents was Berry's integration strategy. Marginalization was least favoured by all groups. Ethnic identity scores were high for all groups and were positively related to life satisfaction for all ethnic groups. Majority identity was important for all groups, but ethnic identity was more important than majority identity for all groups. There was a significant relationship between high ethnic identity scores and psychological adaptation, as measured by mastery and life satisfaction (Robinson, 2003).

Mixed parentage children and young people

This section will explore issues related to identity formation among mixed parentage children and adolescents. The terms 'mixed parentage', 'mixed race', 'dual heritage', and 'biracial' are often used to describe first generation offspring of parents of different 'races'. They most typically describe individuals of black and white heritage (Sebring, 1985) but are not limited to this combination. In this section the terms will refer to individuals of whom one parent is African Caribbean or Asian (Indian, Pakistani, Bangladeshi) and the other white European.

Identity formation 'is crucial for ethnic minority [mixed parentage] children who face many disparagements to self-esteem from the external world' (Bagley, 1993: 72). As children of mixed parentage increase in the population (see Census, 2001), many will manage to achieve truly integrated identities, while others will experience chronic identity conflicts. This latter group will pose a growing challenge to social work professionals in the 21st century.

The topic of racial/ethnic identity in mixed parentage children has received increasing attention in recent years (e.g. Root, 1992; Tizard and Phoenix, 1993, 2003). This interest has been spurred by demographic trends that indicate a rapid increase in the mixed parentage population and by the acknowledgement that there is little well-defined research and theory in the area. The size of the ethnic minority population was 4.6 million in 2001 or 7.9 per cent of the total population of the United Kingdom. Of the ethnic minority population 15 per cent described their ethnic origin as mixed and about a third of this group was from white and black Caribbean backgrounds (Census, 2001). The experiences of these mixed parentage children will vary, reflecting differences in their class, education and family cultures.

Reviews of the limited research in Britain suggest that few children seemed to experience their situation 'as a painful clash of loyalty between black and white' (Wilson, 1987; Tizard and Phoenix, 1993, 2003). In Tizard and Phoenix's (1993) study most of the children had high self-esteem and positive identities. They found that 'a mixed identity was as likely to be positive as a black identity' (1993: 174) and that 'wanting to be white was the major indicator of a problematic identity for mixed parentage adolescents' (Tizard and Phoenix, 1993: 162). Tizard and Phoenix (2003) reported that children were as likely to identify themselves as 'mixed' as they were 'black'. Even if they were seen as black by others, they experienced themselves as 'mixed'. They note that black self-identification among children of mixed parentage tends to correlate with the degree of politicization on issues of 'race' and racism. Tizard and Phoenix's study also found that despite majority 'white' orientations in terms of friendships, racialized conflict situations produced strong black identifications. There are some mixed parentage children whose experiences give cause for concern. Studies have shown that some mixed parentage adolescents in local authority care exhibit identity confusion and low self-esteem (Banks, 1992; 2002; Barn *et al.*, 1997; Maxime, 1993).

Although mixed-parentage children and youngsters encounter the problems faced by most minorities, they must also figure out how to reconcile the heritages of both parents in a society that categorizes individuals into single groups. Thus, if a person wants to achieve positive biracial identity, he or she has to take in and value both racial parts of himself/herself. However, the development of a healthy biracial identity 'means not only accepting and valuing both [black and white] heritages and being comfortable in both the minority and the majority community, but having the flexibility to accept that others may identify them as minority, majority or biracial' (Pinderhughes, 1995: 81).

Carter (1995) argues that 'a person who is biracial should become grounded in the devalued [black] racial group as a foundation for facilitating the merger of the two racial groups. This is particularly true for racial groups in the United States [and Britain]' (1995: 120). According to Carter, 'when one has first developed a positive Black identity and uses the Black identity as a foundation, it allows incorporation of the White aspect of identity' (1995: 120). In a study of racial identity attitudes of mixed parentage (African Caribbean/white) adolescents in Britain, Fatimilehin (1999) used the RIAS-B scale (Parham and Helms, 1981) to investigate the attitude of these youngsters to their black heritage. Fatimilehin (1999) found that older teenagers were more likely to have positive racial identity attitudes, and a positive relationship was found between racial identity attitudes and self-esteem. However, monoracial models of minority identity development do not address all the issues facing mixed parentage adolescents. For example, Cross's (1978, 1991) model includes rejection of the minority culture followed by rejection of the majority culture, and does not include the possibility of integrating more than one racial/ethnic group identity into one's self. Various authors (e.g. Poston, 1990) have argued that there is a need to develop models of biracial identity development.

Several models of biracial identity development have been proposed (e.g. Jacobs, 1992; Kerwin and Ponterotto, 1995; Root, 1992). These authors questioned the applicability of monoracial identity models to those of biracial heritage. Many of these frameworks demonstrate a similar hierarchy of stages that begin with initial learning about race and ethnicity differences, move to the struggle to find an identity but feeling pressured to choose only one group, and end in achievement of some level of biracial identity where both cultures are accepted and integrated into the person's overall identity. Root (1992, 1996) is the exception here. She describes four different paths that individuals can choose, all of which can lead to a positive biracial existence. Her possible outcomes include choosing the identity assigned by others, identifying with both racial groups, choosing one racial group over the others, and identifying with a new, biracial or multiracial group. Although Root (1992) describes how an individual can be successful with any of these choices, her model, like many of the others, implies that the latter of the solutions is possibly the most beneficial. All of these models differ from Stonequist's (1937) early deficit conceptualization of biracial individuals who suffer marginalized existences because they never live fully in either culture of their background.

In an article that reviewed the theories about mixed parentage identity formation. Kerwin and Ponterotto (1995) outlined the following myths regarding mixed parentage children: the stereotype that biracial children are marginal persons; the myth that mixed parentage individuals must choose to identify with only one group; that mixed parentage children do not want to discuss their racial identity. Important variables to consider with these children are that they may choose one group over the other at different stages of their life (Poston, 1990) and that these choices are often influenced by their social and family situation and exposure, the composition and nature of their peer group, their participation in cultural activities, their physical appearance and language facility, inter-group tolerance, and their self-esteem (Kerwin and Ponterotto, 1995; Stephan, 1992).

Social work implications

Discrimination can have damaging effects on the psychological adjustment and self-esteem of young children and adolescents. In particular, through racial prejudice the black child in Britain and America is subjected to derogatory views and negative self-images projected not only by the media, but also by teachers, parents, and the wider society. Early in life, the child acquires knowledge of how the black person is viewed in society.

Black children are constantly bombarded with images that suggest to them that their race is not the preferred race. Except in the spheres of sport and entertainment, when black children look around them they find few role models with their skin colour with important prestigious positions in this society. They see mainly white models in advertisements and as heroes of stories. There is a lack of positive black role models in the media, especially on television. Even today cartoons still usually portray the savage and the evil as the black man.

According to Barnes:

> Blacks are threatened with the specter of white racism from the cradle to the grave. Yet many escape the worst features of oppression, and many have shown an incredible capacity to survive, achieve, and conform in the face of impossible odds. Nevertheless, all blacks are members of a color caste system in this [American] society and are subjected to ruthless oppression.
>
> (Barnes, 1991: 686)

Racial and ethnic identity development models will help social workers recognize differences between members of the same racial and ethnic group with respect to their racial/ethnic identity. The model 'serves as a useful assessment and diagnostic tool for social workers to gain a greater understanding of their culturally different client' (Sue, 2006: 104). Social workers 'who are familiar with the sequence of stages [in racial and ethnic identity development models] are better able to plan intervention strategies that are most effective for culturally different clients' (Sue, 2006: 104). Robinson's (2000) research highlights the importance of studying the racial identity attitudes of young black people in residential care. The residential care staff found Cross's model extremely useful in therapeutic work with African Caribbean youngsters. Although Robinson's (2000) study indicated that pre-encounter attitudes were not widely endorsed by the adolescents in residential care, residential staff need to be aware that an individual holding pre-encounter attitudes may have yet to experience the sort of encounter that will catch them off guard. Maxime (1993) cites several examples of children in local authority care experiencing encounters that shattered the appropriateness of their current identity and worldview. Individuals in the pre-encounter stage are, according to Cross (1995), 'sitting ducks' for an encounter that may cause them to rethink their positions on blackness. As noted earlier, the immersion-emersion stage encompasses the most sensational aspects of black identity development. The individual at this stage tends to denigrate white people and white culture, exhibiting generally anti-white attitudes. This could be 'painful for white residential workers who suddenly find themselves "under attack" verbally and emotionally' (Maxime, 1993: 178). Black adolescents at the immersion-emersion stage are usually suspicious and hostile toward white professionals. They are likely to regard their own psychological problems as products of oppression and racism. A white care worker or fieldworker will be viewed by the black service user as 'a symbol of the oppressive Establishment' (Sue, 2006: 89). Black adolescents in the immersion-emersion stage will constantly test the sincerity and openness of the white care worker, and be likely to share their problems only with a black worker. However, they may also be anxious that the black practitioner will not meet their own standards of blackness since the black worker's education, training, authority and status all depend on participation in the white world.

Many service providers assume that a black staff member is a better therapeutic match for a black service user than a white practitioner. Yet such an assumption seems questionable if, for example, the black care worker has pre-encounter attitudes where, as noted earlier, racial identity attitudes towards blackness are negative and white culture and society are seen as ideal. Similarly, a black worker at the encounter stage may have confused feelings when working with a black client. Thus an individual's stage of racial identity may have a greater impact on the counseling/therapeutic process than does 'race' per se (Carter, 1995).

In a small qualitative study of the care experiences of young black people, Ince (1998: 46) found that all the participants 'reported racisms at school and within their care setting, having limited or no help from carers or professionals to help with the stress and negative feelings left in the wake of racist behaviour'. Social workers need to assess the impact of prejudice and discriminatory practices on the self-image, self-esteem and identity of young black people and must also be cognizant of their own prejudices. Frequently, a social worker's prejudices, which may be subtle, can interfere with the relationship.

Social workers need to take an active approach in helping black children build positive self-images of themselves. A number of workbooks have been published by Maxime (1987) to help social workers. The aim of one workbook, *Black Like Me*, is 'to assist and enhance in the development of a positive and black identity' (Maxime, 1987: 2). Another workbook (Maxime, 1991), intended for black and white children, describes the contributions black people have made in various fields – for example, medicine, mathematics, technology, arts, sports, etc. In Thoburn *et al.*'s (2000: 135) study one young black man placed with black foster parents 'was very positive about the way in which they had helped him to feel good about himself as a black person'. The following is a quote from this young person: 'The foster parents introduced me to some books like Martin Luther King and Malcolm X. So they set me on the road to learning about my blackness .... I think I would have been confused if I'd gone to a white foster family' (2000: 135).

Social workers and educators must begin as early as pre-school age to expose children regularly to black people in positions of power and authority. In addition, children can be provided positive role models through class trips to environments, activities, and engagements that are controlled, produced, managed, or contributed to by black people. The child should be able to identify and talk about blacks of earlier times and the present.

Comer and Pouissant (1992) propose various ways in which black parents can promote racial pride in their children. They suggest that parents 'can discuss color and race-related issues in a natural way' (1992: 17). Thus, when parents are teaching children about colours and body parts and functions, they can describe the child's arm as 'brown' or 'black'. 'When the question of color arises later, it can be discussed in a positive, relaxed manner because [parents] have not previously ignored or overdramatized it' (1992: 17). Social workers working with black children and adolescents can use the techniques described above in helping black children and youth develop a positive black identity.

It is valuable to show children the contributions black people have made to art, music and science (Banks, 2003). However, the child must first 'begin to develop an acceptance of self before being able to identify with another' (2003: 167).

Parents and social workers must look at the books that children read both at school and at home, and must question and discuss with the children the subliminal messages (for example, witches are black, angels are white). They should also address the biases in the English language. For example, the English language is replete with phrases like 'Black Monday', 'black magic', 'black deed', which further maintains the negative self-image that the children adopt.

As noted earlier, acculturation research (Berry, 1997; Berry and Sam, 1997) documents the stress that results when one cultural group comes in contact with another. Adolescents who are members of second or later generations in Britain and US are likely to be well acquainted with the mainstream culture, but may face conflicting demands due to differences between mainstream values and those of their ethnic culture. The issue they must resolve is the way to combine these competing identities; that is, the extent to which they identify with their ethnic culture and also with the larger society. The issue may be problematic for several reasons, including pressures both from within their ethnic group and from the mainstream culture.

Of greatest practical importance for social workers is the question of how ethnic and majority identities and the resulting identity categories are related to the adaptation of minorities and immigrants. Berry's (1990) acculturation model proposes that immigrants adopting an integration strategy show better psychological adaptation than those favouring the other acculturation orientations (for example, assimilation). In Britain, Robinson (2003) found that the integration strategy related positively and significantly with life satisfaction for Asian and African Caribbean adolescents. Because of the importance of one's ethnic identity as a defining characteristic of minority and immigrant group members (Phinney, 1990), pressures to assimilate and give up one's sense of ethnicity may result in anger, depression, and in some cases violence. Social workers need to be aware that integration, that is, simultaneous ethnic retention and adaptation to the new society, is the most adaptive mode of acculturation and the most conducive to immigrant and minority adolescents' well-being, whereas marginalization is the worst (Berry, 1997; Berry and Sam, 1997).

The increase in the number of mixed parentage children in care (Department of Health, 2001) poses a new set of challenges for social workers. It will be necessary for social workers to expand their knowledge in this area through continued education, workshops and in-service training. Social workers need to be aware of their own opinions and biases about interracial marriages, racial identity of biracial persons, and their own personal identity, and be aware of internalized racial and ethnic stereotypes.

In a small scale study of children of mixed heritage in need in Islington, Sinclair and Hai (2002: 33) note that 'the quality of information on children's background needs to be improved; more detail is needed on … all aspects of ethnicity – "race", culture, religion and language'. Social workers need to ensure that 'carers are adequately prepared and supported in helping children develop and sustain a positive self image and to understand their full ethnic background' (Sinclair and Hai, 2002: 33). The young people in Sinclair and Hai's (2002) study indicated a positive awareness of their ethnicity. However, there was still recognition that this did give rise to particular needs: about accepting all aspects of their heritage, especially from an absent parent; and about addressing racism, sometimes from within the family. The authors report that both social workers and carers were active in addressing these needs, for example, 'by trying to maintain some "quality" contact with the different aspects of the child's background, through engagement with the local "ethnic" communities … and using of cultural activities to foster positive contact' (2002: 34).

Prevatt-Goldstein and Spencer (2000) suggest the following principles for social workers finding suitable placements for mixed parentage children: 'ensuring that the child … develops those heritages that are most minimized or devalued [and] ensuring that the valuing and reflection of these heritages does not diminish the promotion of, or access to, other identities of the child' (2000: 14).

Finally, I wish to mention the practice of transracial adoption. This is a controversial area of social work practice (for a full discussion, see Bagley, 1993; Small, 1984, 1986; Treacher and Katz, 2000). Maxime argued that 'Black children growing up in white families fail to develop a positive black identity. Instead, they suffer identity confusion and develop a negative self-concept, believing or wishing that they were white, and harbouring negative attitudes towards black people' (Maxime, 1986: 101). Small asserts that: 'unless they are very carefully trained, white families cannot provide black children with the skills and "survival techniques" they need for coping in a racist society' (Small, 1986: 85). The Association of Black Social Workers and Allied Professions has also attacked the practice of transracial placements in Britain (ABSWAP, 1983). Tizard and Phoenix do not agree with the psychological objections to transracial adoptions as they maintain that these objections 'are not well grounded in either empirical data or theory' (2003: 67). According to Zeitlin (2002: 248) 'the pessimism over placement of children with physically dissimilar families – "transracial" adoptions – is unjustified and the majority do well'. However, social workers should make an effort to recruit more black families.

Various authors (for example, Maxime, 1986, 1997; Small, 1984), including myself, prefer same-race placements. However, if social workers have to place black children in white homes, they must ensure that transracial adoptees be raised in racially aware contexts. In such a context the family acknowledges and accepts the child's race. The families usually live in racially diverse neighborhoods, and the children attend integrated schools. Typically, adoptees are familiarized and even actively involved with their birth cultures. Adoptees raised in such a context are more likely to develop positive racial identities (Andujo, 1988; DeBerry, 1991; McRoy *et al.*, 1984; Kallgren and Caudill, 1993: 552).

For black American adolescents adopted by white parents, McRoy and Zurcher found that 'the opportunity for establishing positive relationships with blacks on an everyday basis was a key factor in the child's development of a positive black identity and a corresponding feeling about other blacks' (1983: 134).

Much more must be written, researched, and published in order that all of us may better understand what experiences are necessary and therefore should be provided to every black child and adult in order to facilitate the development of a positive black identity. Social workers still have much work ahead in the area of fostering healthy, positive, self-images in black children and adolescents.

6 Educational achievement and the black child

Introduction

The black perspectives on issues critical to the educational achievement of black children are presented in this chapter. It will introduce the reader to the perspectives of black social scientists on matters related to the educational achievement of blacks. I believe that it is incumbent upon black social scientists to carefully evaluate research and writing in the area of educational achievement and to put forward the black perspectives. This chapter attempts to meet this objective.

The deficit approach

A review of the literature on the major issues involved in testing black children reveals two general models – a 'deficit' and a 'difference' model. The deficit approach assumes that black people are deficient when compared to whites in some measurable trait called intelligence, and that this deficiency is due to genetic or cultural factors or both. This approach has reinforced stereotypes that characterized black people as inferior, and has maintained the comparatively low teacher expectations that produce academic underachievement.

Early explanations for lower academic and intellectual functioning among black children referred to 'genetic deficits' in the black population. The theories, findings, and conclusions produced by many Euro-American psychologists have been used to try to demonstrate that blacks are mentally inferior to whites. For example, the conclusions of leading psychologists such as Edward Thorndike, Lewis Terman and Arthur Jensen regarding the innate mental inferiority of blacks, were considered respectable and generally accepted in the social scientific community (discussed in Chapter 1). Jensen (1969), for example, claims that blacks, as a group, tend to score significantly less (about

15 IQ points) than whites on intelligence tests. The research and writing about black-white differences in intelligence has generated a great deal of controversy (see Williams and Mitchell, 1981). Hilliard (1981) described intelligence testing as having questionable validity and purpose, and no practical application to instruction. One of the most widely used tests for the measurement of children's intelligence, the Wechsler Intelligence Scale for Children-Revised (WISC-R), is considered to be an extremely biased and limited test by many black educators and psychologists (Hilliard, 1987). As there are numerous definitions of intelligence, 'each test developer makes a subjective decision about what "intelligence" will mean for his test' (Williams *et al.*, 2004: 466). On this point, Chaplin states that:

> In spite of the prevalence of intelligence testing, psychologists have found it difficult to define intelligence precisely ... most of the psychologists who developed the early tests side-stepped the problem of the precise nature of what they were measuring and attempted to make their scales good predictors of scholastic achievement ... most psychologists think of intelligence in much the same way that physicists think of time. Time is what chronometers measure. By the same logic, intelligence is what tests measure.
>
> (Chaplin, 1975: 263–4).

If a test is made specifically for a particular group one would expect members of that group to score higher on the test than members from out-groups. Most standardized IQ (intelligence quotient) tests in use today are culture-specific in that they are composed of items and validated against responses taken from the specific culture of the white middle class. Hence, persons belonging to other socio-economic classes and other racial groups tend to make responses that deviate from the identified norm. Wilson asserts that:

> The 'intelligence' determined by IQ tests is the 'intelligence' which may be defined as the degree to which an individual has assimilated and accommodated, i.e., adapted, himself to a certain set of values, standards, attitudes, ways of verbalizing, ways of thinking, ways of perceiving and other ways of behaving that a particular culture, subculture or individual evaluates as important to the maintenance and advancement of its way of life. Thus, intelligence is always culturally or individually defined.
>
> (Wilson, 1978: 134)

It appears that 'the minority individual is being judged by a test which is based on an experience which he [or she] has not been allowed to have and which gives no credibility to his [or her] actual experiences' (Williams *et al.*, 2004: 467). The black child has 'to be virtually "white", at least in the cognitive-behaviour sense if not in the full cultural sense' (Wilson, 1978: 132) in order to achieve a high score on IQ tests. Black people have to 'become "white" before their talents and cognitive functions are permitted full and free expression' (Wilson, 1978: 132). It is evident that the Eurocentric cultural paradigm which guides the assessment and evaluation of reality stands in contradistinction to the cultural laws of African people (Nobles, 1986).

As a means of correcting for this bias, some investigators have suggested that separate intelligence tests should be developed for minority groups. In 1972, Williams developed the Black Intelligence Test of Cultural Homogeneity. As we have seen in Chapter 1, this test is specific to black (African-American) culture and consists of material that is unfamiliar to most middle-class whites. The Williams test is a 100-item, multiple choice test consisting of words and phrases taken from the black experience. Though not yielding an actual IQ, the results are helpful in determining the degree of an individual's familiarity with black values, traditions, customs, and overall worldview, as reflected in the vocabulary of black culture. Blacks score consistently higher than whites on black culture-specific tests (Williams *et al.*, 2004).

Psychologists have attempted to develop a 'culture free' test, which would represent 'an attempt at stripping the individual of his cultural veneer in order to reveal and expose his true and inherent abilities' (Samuda, 1975: 133). However, after some attempts, investigators recognized that 'a culture-free test was simply an impossibility' (Samuda, 1975: 133), and the focus shifted to the development of 'culture-fair' tests. Wilson maintains that 'culture-fair' tests are not 'free of [their] cultural roots ... for they still test cognitive-behavioral-perceptual patterns that are deemed important by a culture or test-maker' (Wilson, 1978: 134). He goes on to state that: 'No test, IQ or otherwise, has been found or created that determines the true intellectual capacity of an individual' (1978: 134).

Shade has also addressed the problem of 'culture-fair' tests. Her research findings – that blacks (African Americans) interpret visual images differently than whites – have major implications for tests, including so-called 'culture-fair' tests, that involve analysing visual information or completing visual perception tasks (Shade, 1991). Shade asserts that:

For each of these instruments [tests], a less than expected performance by African Americans has been interpreted as a deficit .... [However] a more plausible explanation may be that African Americans have merely been taught to perceive, that is, to visually transform, the world differently.

(Shade, 1991: 242)

The cultural deprivation model focused on the 'environmental handicaps' confronting black families and children (e.g. Moynihan, 1965). It was argued that economic and social discrimination led to self-perpetuating conditions that resulted in the development of dysfunctional personality traits (e.g. low self-concept and a low need for achievement) which resulted in lower achievement levels among black children. The problem with the cultural deprivation model is that it continued to 'blame the victim' (see Ryan, 1967) by pointing to 'pathological families' and a 'culture of poverty' (see Baratz and Baratz, 1970; Bernard, 2001; Valentine, 1971).

Current IQ test debates

Perhaps the most profound challenge to IQ thinking and testing comes from a spate of recent studies that document, in a clear way, the importance of well organized regular education (Hilliard, 2004). For example, in one study, 'Saunders and Rivers (1998) showed that the simple practice of giving students three good teachers in a row resulted in 50 percentile ranks of difference between the IQ means of these children and those who got three bad teachers in a row' (Hilliard, 2004: 274).

The IQ testing debate should have ended before the 1990s (Hayles *et al.*, 2004). Nonetheless, in 1994, Hernstein and Murray's book – *The Bell Curve* – rekindled the debate (see Hernstein and Murray, 1994 for detailed review). These authors provided data to suggest that intelligence differs among racial groups and that black people are at the lowest end of the bell curve. A major point of the book is that most social problems, especially those found among economically and socially marginalized people, can not be solved because they are linked to intelligence, which is mainly inherited. Therefore, environmental supports put in place to solve these problems will not be useful if the social problem is due to intelligence. *The Bell Curve* has been subject to intense scrutiny and criticism because of its erroneous assumptions and methodological flaws (Yee *et al.*, 1993; Haynes, 1995).

An excellent critique of *The Bell Curve* was provided by Haynes, 1995. Not only did racial bias and questionable methodologies plague work pertaining to IQ, but the alleged IQ difference between blacks and whites did not appear to be present at birth as previously hypothesized (Haynes, 1995). In fact, in another critique of Hernstein and Murray's work, Madhere (1995) offered a 'metabolic model' of talent and character development. This model suggested that academic failure or underachievement denote discontinuity in the learning experiences of some urban African American learners within the American educational system. Madhere disputed the claims that intelligence is unidimensional and immutable and that the source of differences between racial groups are rooted in intellectual abilities. Madhere noted that *The Bell Curve* authors deliberately ignored advances made in the study of intelligence (see Madhere, 1995 for a review). According to Donovan and Cross:

> No contemporary test author or publisher endorses the notion that IQ tests are direct measures of innate ability. Yet misconceptions that the tests reflect genetically determined, innate ability that is fixed throughout the life span remain prominent with the public, many educators, and some social scientists.
>
> (Donovan and Cross, 2002: 284).

In recent years, research on intelligence has developed. According to Gardner (1993) individuals have multiple intelligences. These include: (1) verbal; (2) mathematical; (3) spatial; (4) kinaesthetic; (5) musical; (6) interpersonal; and (7) intrapsychic intelligences. In general, these intelligences are changeable. Since 1993, others have expanded the list to include other factors. Notably, emotional intelligence has been added (Hayles *et al.*, 2004: 408).

The difference model

In contrast to the cultural deprivation model, the cultural difference model strongly rejects the assumptions of the cultural deficit theorists, and argues that differences noted by psychologists in intelligence testing, behaviours, lifestyles, languages, etc. can be judged as appropriate or inappropriate only within a specific cultural context (White, 1972, 2004). Thus, to say that the black child is different from the white child is not to say that he/she is inferior, deficient, or deprived. The difference model acknowledges that each culture has strengths and limitations, and, rather than being labelled as deficient, differences between ethnic groups are regarded as simply different. A person can be unique and different without being labelled inferior. Differences between black and white groups 'in language and dialect may produce differences in cognitive learning styles, but a difference is not a deficiency' (Williams, 1972: 82). Therefore:

> Instead of calling black language wrong, improper, or deficient in nature, one must realize that the black child is speaking a well-developed language commonly referred to as non-standard English. Intelligence is frequently based quite heavily on language factors. It is a common observation that black and white children do not speak alike. The differences in linguistic systems favor white children since standard English is the 'lingua franca' of the tests.
>
> (Williams, 1972: 82)

White also points out that white researchers or educational psychologists 'listening to black speech assume that ... [black people's] use of nonstandard oral English is an example of bad grammar without recognizing the possibility that ... [black people] have a valid, legitimate, alternate dialect' (2004: 6).

Compensatory education programmes (for example, Head Start) were set up to 'provide black children with the kind of enrichment ... [the white psychologist] feels is needed to overcome and compensate for their cultural deprivation' (White, 2004: 6). These programmes failed, as they were based on the assumptions, goals, and methods of cultural deprivation theorists (Banks, 1982). What is needed is for psychologists and educators to 'stop trying to compensate for the so-called weaknesses of the black child, and try to develop a theory that capitalizes on his strengths' (White, 2004: 6). A black perspective rejects the 'deficit theory' when explaining cultural group differences in intellectual performance. The educational system must recognize black children's strengths, abilities, and culture and incorporate them into the learning process.

Antecedents of educational achievement

A discussion of the antecedents of educational achievement will be preceded by a summary of the data on the academic achievement of black children. I do not intend to present data from, or even to summarize, all the British studies in the field of educational achievement and ethnicity. Those readers who wish to obtain some overview of this field should consult Casen and Kingdon (2007), Tomlinson (1983, 2005), Taylor and Hegarty (1986), Gillborn (1990), Modood (2005).

Over the past thirty years the educational achievement of black children and young people in Britain has attracted an enormous amount of research. Kelly maintains that:

> The findings are not totally consistent, but the general conclusion is that children of West Indian origin under-achieve in British schools, even compared to inner-city whites. West Indian boys do particularly badly. On the other hand children of Asian origin seem to achieve as well as comparable whites, especially when they have been in Britain for some time.
>
> (Kelly, 1988: 113)

Research evidence over the last few decades has consistently shown some young people, notably African Caribbean, Pakistani and Bangladeshi, to under-achieve in schools (Modood, 2005; Tomlinson, 2005). Underachievement among African Caribbean, Pakistani and Bangladeshi pupils continues at GCSE level. In contrast, Chinese and Indian pupils do very well, outperforming other pupils. African Caribbean pupils are among the least successful ethnic groups by the time they reach 16 years of age. They are four times more likely to be excluded from secondary school and considerably less likely to get five or more GCSE passes at grades A to C (Majors *et al.*, 2001).

In a recent study, Cassen and Kingdon (2007) found that while 'Chinese and Indian pupils are the most successful in avoiding low achievement; Afro-Caribbean pupils are the least successful on average .... Bangladeshi, Pakistani and Black African are among those not achieving any passes above [grade] D' (Cassen and Kingdon, 2007: 8). Gilborn and Mirza (2000) argue that although information about differential achievement and ethnicity is important in understanding inequalities in educational outcomes, care should be taken to avoid a racially hierarchical view based on assumptions of inherent ability.

Levels of achievement among black African Caribbeans have been a focus of attention at both national and local level. According to Mabey (1986: 173), 'much of the research on black pupils' achievement has suggested either explicitly or implicitly that the causes lie in the individuals themselves'. The cultural deficit arguments adopted by Daniel Moynihan (1965) and others in the USA have shown remarkable resilience and continue to surface in the debate about the differential performance of students of Asian and African-Caribbean origin in school.

The explanations put forward by the Swann Committee (1985) for the differential school performances of Asians and African Caribbeans will serve to illustrate the deficit argument. In 1978, the British government set up a committee of inquiry into the education of ethnic minority pupils. The committee was asked to focus initially on factors influencing the educational attainments of young people of 'West Indian' origin because of fears that their continuing poor academic performance would precipitate 'alienation', 'disillusionment', and ultimately violent outbreaks in major urban areas (see Troyna, 1984; Troyna and Williams, 1986, for elaboration). With Anthony Rampton as its chairman the committee produced an interim report in 1981 which corroborated the conventional view that pupils of West Indian origin were 'underfunctioning' in school compared to their 'Asian' and 'White' peers. Four years later, now with Lord Swann as the chairman, the committee produced its final report, *Education for All* (or the Swann report as it is generally known) which confirmed this trend. That is, pupils of 'West Indian' origin do less well than their white counterparts in school examinations. The Swann Committee of Inquiry concluded that 'West Indian children as a group are underachieving in our education system and this should be a matter of deep concern not only to all those involved in education but also the whole community' (Swan, 1985). 'Asians' on the other hand, often do as well as 'whites' and sometimes perform even better (Swan, 1985; see also Chivers, 1987). The Swann Committee noted that 'the reasons for the very different school performances of Asians and West Indians seem likely to lie within their respective cultures' (1985: 87). As indicated above, it is evident that this explanation resembles the cultural deficit – or 'blaming the victim' – theory and is similar to the one proposed by Moynihan (1965) of the 'Negro' family in the 1960s. It appears that the cultural deficit theory retains a firm grip on educational research and policy initiatives in Britain. More recent studies have contradicted the earlier pattern of Asian success and African-Caribbean failure, as suggested by Kelly (1988). Thus:

> Current research has indicated quite clearly that relating ethnic categories to educational success and failure had not fully indicated the complex patterns of underachievement manifest amongst the minority communities (Tanna, 1990). Recently, it has become evident that some children of particular Asian backgrounds are at the very bottom of the performance league (DES, 1985; CRE, 1990).
>
> (Lashley and Pumfrey, 1993: 118)

There is evidence to suggest that African-Caribbean students have been over-represented in special education provision (Majors, 2001). Ely and

Denny suggest that 'differences between Asian and West Indian under-performance may well be linked to the higher number of Asians with middle class backgrounds' (Ely and Denny, 1989: 56). According to Modood (2005) the better performance of Asians could be due to their values which emphasise education and encourage social mobility.

The educational achievement of children from different ethnic backgrounds and the factors which affect their achievement continue to attract attention. Many different explanations have been put forward by researchers attempting to discover causal factors behind differential levels of achievement between white and black pupils in both the UK and the US. Bagley, Bart, and Wong (1979) noted that there had been little research emphasis, either in the USA or Britain, on why some black children succeed in school. The authors point out that 'such a research strategy ... offers much insight into why some, but not all, blacks may underachieve. It offers, too, practical avenues of educational and social policy for enhancing black achievement' (Bagley, Bart and Wong, 1979: 84). In fact 'the possibility of acknowledging black achievement seems problematic to those wishing to assert simplistic models of race, culture and underachievement' (Mirza, 1992: 193). Identifying the antecedents of academic achievement for black children and youth has been the focus of several studies.

Gillborn and Gipps (1996) argue that the negative school experiences of some African Caribbean boys appear to be an important element in their academic under-achievement. They highlight lack of fluency in English as one significant factor leading to the early under-achievement of Pakistani and Bangladeshi pupils. However, given that research informs us that other pupils with early fluency difficulties do make substantial progress, it is not clear why Pakistani and Bangladeshi pupils perform poorly at GCSE level. Cassen and Kingdon (2007: 1) found that 'not speaking English at home is typically a short-lived handicap ... Asian students who experience it commonly recover by secondary school'. Luthra (1997) believes that the research into comparative under-achievement, as opposed to relative progression, has led to a 'victimology of its own thus catalyzing the culture of failure within the same groups'.

Many factors have been identified in the literature in explaining the differential academic success of black children but some of the more common factors include: the self-concept, teacher expectation, and family disposition (Majors, 2001; Osborne, 2001; Tomlinson, 1983; Verma and Ashworth, 1986; Verma and Pumfrey, 1988; Clark, 1983).

Black self-concept

Before proceeding with this discussion I wish to stress that I am opposed to attributing the problems black people face in education to any psychological deficiencies. This would be akin to 'the theories "liberal" social scientists have used to blame victims for their plights (Ryan, 1971; Baratz and Baratz, 1970)' (Burlew, 1979: 165). Nevertheless, the low expectations black people might harbour about achieving educational goals 'would be the natural reaction of any group with an oppressed history and an unfavourable position in the current social structure' (Burlew, 1979: 166).

One factor identified in the literature as contributing to or preventing the academic achievement of black children is the self-concept (some aspects of the self-concept have been discussed in Chapter 5). Both British and American studies 'have put forward the view that self-esteem is a determinant of educational achievement' (Verma and Ashworth, 1986: 36). Nevertheless, there are disputable answers to the question of how the self-concept impacts on achievement aspirations. It has been argued by psychologists and sociologists (for example, Mead, 1934; Cooley, 1956) that the self arises through the individual's interaction with and reaction to other members of society: his/her peers, parents, and teachers. The collective attitudes of the others, the community or 'generalized other' as Mead calls them, give the individual his/her unity of self. The individual's self is shaped, developed, and controlled by his/her anticipating and assuming the attitudes and definitions of others (the community) towards him/her. Cooley suggested that the self was like the looking-glass which mirrored the three principal components of one's self-concept: 'the imagination of our appearance to the other person; the imagination of his judgement of that appearance; and some sort of self-feeling, such as pride or mortification' (Cooley, 1956: 50).

For black children in white British or American society, the generalized other whose attitudes he/she assumes and the looking-glass into which he/she gazes both reflect the same judgement: he/she is inferior because he/she is black. (The looking-glass of white society also reflects the supposed undesirability of the black youth's physical appearance, as opposed to the valued models of white physical characteristics.) Alvin Pouissant suggests that:

> Black [African-American] children, like all children, come into the world victims of factors over which they have no control. In the looking glass of white society, the supposedly undesirable physical image of 'Tar Baby' – black skin, wooly hair and thick lips – is

contrasted unfavorably with the valued model of 'Snow White' – white skin, straight hair and aquiline features.

(Pouissant, 1974: 138)

If the concept of necessary external validation is accurate, it seems reasonable to assume that the achievement aspirations of black children would be influenced by evaluations by significant others in the child's life. While such an assertion might be reasonable, researchers have had difficulty agreeing on whence the child's source of validation is derived. Some research suggests that validation and approval are derived from the black community (Banks and Grambs, 1972; Barnes, 1972; Norton, 1983). However, the larger body of research suggests that approval is sought from the dominant white culture (Kardiner and Ovessey, 1951); and, because of the negative attitudes perpetuated by the larger white society, positive achievement by blacks was not an expected outcome. Coombs and Davies offer the important proposition that:

> In the context of the school world, a student who is defined as a 'poor student' (by significant others and thereby by self) comes to conceive of himself [herself] as such and gears his [her] behaviour accordingly, that is, the social expectation is realized. However, if he [she] is led to believe by means of the social 'looking glass' that he [she] is capable and able to achieve well, he [she] does. To maintain his [her] status and self-esteem becomes the incentive for further effort which subsequently involves him [her] more in the reward system of the school.
>
> (Coombs and Davies, 1966: 468–9)

Studies of the black self-concept and self-esteem have generally assumed that every aspect of black life is a reflection of the group's (subordinate) position in the dominant white society, and that black people are not capable of rejecting the negative images of themselves perpetuated by the dominant white society. Research carried out as early as 1939 by Clark and Clark (discussed in Chapter 5) documented the negative and confused racial attitudes frequently expressed by black children. The black children who participated in the Clarks' studies usually expressed a preference for white dolls and rejected the black dolls. The authors concluded that the children's choice of white dolls was a reflection of their group self-hatred. Research conducted by Goodman (1952) and Morland (1958) confirmed the Clark findings. They found that black children under five frequently manifested uneasiness because of their awareness of skin differences. Morland showed kindergarten children pictures of black and white children and asked them which children they preferred as playmates. The study showed a preference for whites as expressed by the majority of subjects. This research indicates that preference for whites by children of both races developed early, even before racial differences could be communicated. The literature suggested that these identity problems were linked to problems of self-evaluation.

In a study of black adolescents, Spencer, Noll, Stoltzfus and Harpalani (2001) found that youngsters who were at Cross's (1971, 1991) Pre-Encounter stage (see Chapter 5), showed lower academic achievement and lower self-esteem than those pupils who were at the Internalization stage. The study indicates that 'a strong, proactive sense of Black cultural identity is associated with positive academic achievement for Black youth' (Spencer and Harpalani, 2006: 1).

Both American and British studies of self-esteem among black pupils have produced contradictory findings. Bagley, Mallick, and Verma's study (1979) revealed that differences in self-esteem between African Caribbeans and whites existed only for boys; there were no differences between the African-Caribbean girls and their white counterparts. Other British studies (Driver, 1980; Louden, 1978; Stone, 1985) have reported higher self-esteem among black pupils, and particularly the girls. The British studies have tended to concentrate on African-Caribbean pupils. In the same study cited above, Louden (1978) found that Asian pupils had higher levels of self-esteem than either African-Caribbean or white pupils. Many authors have challenged the self-concept theorists' notion of negative black self-esteem. American research (Powell and Fuller, 1970) cites evidence that black children develop a greater self-esteem than shown in previous findings, and prefer people of their own colour to whites. Black children do not believe or agree with negative stereotypes about themselves or that they are inferior (Brigham, 1974; Rosenberg, 1979). Literature reviews (for example, Wylie, 1978; Rosenberg, 1979) and studies (Dukes and Martinez, 1994; Morgan, 1995) showed little or no differences in self-concept between black and white children, and higher self-esteem scores in black children. Jones (2004) suggests that recent studies have shown that while the self-esteem levels of black people now are at least as high as those of whites, the average academic attainment among African American students is still below that of whites. They conclude that the evidence appears to show quite conclusively that the low self-esteem hypothesis is neither a necessary nor sufficient explanation of African American achievement levels.

Despite the contradictory findings on studies of the black child's self-concept, there appears to be general agreement among scholars that a child's sense of self influences his or her academic achievement (for example, Bagley, Mallick and Verma, 1979; Driver, 1982; Majors, 2001). However, we must be careful not to conclude that black under-achievement is only 'the result of a widespread problem of low self esteem' (German, 2002: 205). According to Verma and Ashworth: 'Self-esteem ... offers another angle on educational achievement ... it can provide another dimension of the factors mediating on achievement' (Verma and Ashworth, 1986: 37).

Gibson (1986) suggests that a major causal factor in the under-achievement of African-Caribbean pupils at school and at work is stress:

> [T]he stress of living in a society that devalues them because of their skin colour. Among the debilitating symptoms of this condition are a lack of confidence and self-esteem, poor sense of aspiration, low breaking-point and an inability to cope with the challenges and demands of their situation in Britain.
>
> (Gibson, 1986: 93)

German (2002: 205) points out that 'the trigger to racial violence and discrimination is skin colour ...'.

Other British studies have also indicated that self-esteem is signifi-cantly related to academic achievement for 'disadvantaged' as well as other pupils (Coard, 1971; Milner, 1975). If this is true, one must ask what all those professionals (e.g. teachers, social workers), who work closely with black children can do to promote the development of a positive self-concept (see Chapter 5). German (2002) states that a

> positive sense of identity is enhanced by the presence of role mod-els, relevant curriculum content and resources that provide positive images of black children, but one needs to remember that racial violence and discrimination do not avoid choosing as their victims black children and adults who are self-aware, self-confident and assertive.
>
> German (2002: 205)

In Britain, the self-concept theorists were influential in guiding the multi-cultural education debate. As a result, changes in the curriculum were proposed to strengthen the self-esteem of black pupils. Black children can hardly avoid developing a deep sense of inferiority and worthlessness if they are constantly fed on an ethnocentric curriculum that presents their communities and cultures in a highly biased and unflattering manner. Making the curriculum more culturally relevant with exposure to history, culture, heroes, and symbols helps students believe in the possibilities and potentialities for them to achieve. Textbooks and curriculum guides that are used every day in the classroom should, at a minimum, contain figures that mirror the experiences of black students in their communities. However, multicultural and anti-racist education has 'proved to be little more than rhetoric, and has been perceived to be ill thought out, [and] piecemeal ...' (Barn, 2001: 40). Tomlinson (2005) points out that 'Failure to develop a curriculum for a multiethnic society has contributed to an increase in xenophobia and racism'.

It is important to recognize that motivation to learn is enhanced when students see the need, relevance, and reason for each lesson they learn. Educators should be encouraged to design their lesson plans around resolving contemporary issues that students must confront in their day-to-day lives (Majors, 2001). It is also necessary to 'bring more black role models into the educational arena as practitioners and managers' (White and Johnson, 1972: 279). They continue: 'We must begin to help educational technocrats see the value of and utilize the experience bases which black children and youth bring to schooling' (1972: 280).

Teacher expectations

Teachers' negative attitudes, stereotyped views, and low expectations are a major factor in explaining the academic achievement of the black child. Teacher expectations can serve a self-fulfilling prophecy. Such a possibility was demonstrated by the research of Rosenthal and Jacobson (1968) in their now classic study *Pygmalion in the Classroom*. (Most of the studies suggesting that teacher attitudes and expectations affect a child's performance appeared in the late 1960s and early 1970s.) The methods and conclusions of Rosenthal and Jacobson are by now well known and hence can be summarized briefly. The study predicted that teachers' expectations would significantly affect the learning of a group of primary school children, when their teachers were told the children possessed special intellectual talents. The teachers were also told that these 'talented' children would show marked intellectual improvement by the end of the first few months of the study. In fact, the study demonstrated that the intellectually 'talented' children scored significantly higher than the control group on measures of IQ (47 per cent of the 'talented' children gained 20 or more total IQ points). Rosenthal and Jacobson explained their findings by suggesting that teachers pay more attention to children who are expected to show intellectual promise. These children are often treated in a more encouraging manner, and teachers tend to show increased tolerance and patience with the child's learning process. The opposite is true for children labelled as less intellectually gifted. Thus, when children are not expected to make significant educational gains, then less attention and encouragement are given to them. The Rosenthal studies have been criticized on many methodological grounds (Thorndike, 1968). However, the results of related investigations (for example, Beez, 1969; Palardy, 1969; Pidgeon, 1970; Rubovitz and Maehr, 1973; Watt *et al.*, 1999), suggest that teachers do hold low expectations for certain groups of students and that such expectations do relate to the ways in which teachers interact with their pupils. In the study by Beez (1969), for example, the sample comprised sixty teachers and sixty pupils in a Head Start scheme. Teachers taught each child the meaning of a symbol. Half the teachers had been given the expectancy that, based on a psychological appraisal of the child, good learning would occur; the remaining half were led to expect poor learning. The results were in the predicted direction. Seventy-seven per cent of those alleged to have good intellectual prospects learned five or more symbols, whereas only 13 per cent of those alleged to have poor prospects achieved at this level. Moreover, teachers who had been given favourable expectations about their pupils actually attempted to teach more symbols than those teachers who had been given unfavourable expectations about their pupils. Beez (1969) proposed that the differences in performance among the pupils were partly due to the expectations of the pupils held by teachers of both groups.

In another study, Palardy (1969) examined the differential perceptions of teachers and the different effects these perceptions would have on boys and girls learning to read. Palardy found that when boys were taught by teachers who perceived their ability to learn to be as good as girls, boys learned as well as girls. However, when the boys were taught by teachers who perceived their ability to learn to be lower than girls, boys were outperformed by girls. When black and white males are compared, teachers tend to predict higher test results for white males than they do for black males (Irvine, 1990). Teachers' assessments of black pupils are in fact consistently lower than their actual test results (OFSTED, 1999). Wrench and Hassan (1996) found that African Caribbean males felt that teachers often had negative views of them. Indeed, 'not only were black boys negatively stereotyped by teachers, but also feared by them' (Majors, 2001: 5).

Several studies have found that teachers tend to like pupils who live up (or down) to their expectations regardless of whether those expectations are positive or negative (Blanck, 1993; Rubovitz and

Maehr, 1973). In a study conducted by Rubovitz and Maehr, for example, the differential expectations of white teachers with respect to students' race and learning ability were examined. A group of four mixed-ability eighth grade pupils (two black African Americans and two whites) were allocated to one of sixty-six white women teachers (creating sixty-six teacher-pupil groupings), and two of the four students in each group (one African-American and one white) were randomly given high IQ scores. Rubovitz and Maehr (1973) found differential teacher expectancy effects in predicted directions, and the students' race proved to be a salient factor. Both 'gifted' and 'nongifted' blacks received less favourable treatment than 'gifted' and 'nongifted' whites. The teachers were found to treat black pupils less positively, ignoring them more in class, praising them less and criticizing them more than white pupils. The teachers gave increased attention and encouragement to gifted whites followed by nongifted whites, nongifted blacks, and gifted blacks. Essentially, black giftedness was punished with less attention and praise, whereas white giftedness was rewarded. Teachers who tended to stereotype blacks showed the most negative patterns in teaching black pupils. Because of the lower expectations held by teachers for black pupils, it can be seen that a pupil will often be rewarded (liked) for failure and punished (disliked) for success. In a similar British study Rubovitz and Maehr (1973), Green (1982) demonstrated that 'intolerant' teachers gave least time and attention in class to African-Caribbean boys and Asian girls. These studies demonstrate that teacher expectations have a significant effect on black children's school achievement. Low expectations by teachers usually lead to a self-fulfilling prophecy cycle of failure by the pupils. Low teacher expectation can strongly influence the decline in academic motivation among black students, particularly in the higher classes (Hill, 1999; Stevenson and Davis, 2004). Some black/African American parents, particularly those whose children attend poor, inner city schools, become discouraged by the racism inherent in the self-fulfilling prophecies and withdraw from active involvement in their children's schools; others become so angry in meetings that they alienate teachers (Boyd-Franklin, 2003: 157).

In Britain, there has been growing concern about the educational underachievement of pupils from certain ethnic minority groups, most notably African-Caribbean students (Osborne, 2001). In explaining this phenomenon, increasing prominence has been given to teacher expectations (Gillborn, 2001). The early work of Pidgeon (1970) in Britain supported the conclusion that teacher expectations of pupils are a significant factor in their subsequent achievement. It has been suggested that certain teachers have unfavourable views of African-

Caribbean pupils and perceive them in a negative light. In a booklet entitled *How the West Indian Child is Made ESN in the British School System*, Bernard Coard (1971) argues that teachers' attitudes and expectations towards black (African-Caribbean) children has caused them to underestimate the ability of all black children. Coard (1971) quoted teachers who were not willing to put pressure on the black child, as they felt that the black child was not able to cope academically. The reports of the Committee of Inquiry into the Education of Children from Ethnic Minority Groups (Swann, 1985) argued that teachers' expectations were an important influence on the achievement of African-Caribbean children. It stated:

> we find ourselves all the more convinced of the major role which the particular expectations and attitudes which many teachers have, not only of West Indian pupils, but indeed of pupils from the whole range of ethnic minority groups, can and do play in the educational experience and perhaps the academic achievement of these pupils ... research findings and our own evidence have indicated that the stereotypes that teachers tend to have of West Indian children are often related to a particular and generally negative, expectation of academic performance.
>
> (Swann, 1985: 25)

Short argues that, in Britain, there is 'no conclusive evidence to confirm the allegation that many teachers, as a result of their socialization, subscribe to negative stereotypes of West Indian children, or that they respond to these children in ways that convey a negative stereotype' (Short, 1985: 100). However, in another study of teacher attitudes, Wright (1986) found that a number of teachers in two comprehensive schools in the Midlands held negative and hostile attitudes to their African-Caribbean students. In a later study, Mac an Ghaill (1988) found that many of the teachers in an inner-city secondary school exhibited negative, stereotyped attitudes towards African-Caribbean students in staffroom conversations and interviews. Mac an Ghaill found that 'Afro-Caribbean male students tended to be seen as having "low ability" and potential discipline problems' (Mac an Ghaill, 1988: 64). In a study of black female pupils, Mirza found that 'it was not uncommon to find teachers expressing openly their misgivings about the intellectual capabilities of the black girls in their care' (Mirza, 1992: 53). In fact, '75 per cent of the teachers in the study made at least one negative comment about the black girls they taught' (Mirza, 1992: 53). Although the girls in the study were:

> Aware of their teachers' negative attitudes towards them ... there
> was little evidence that they [the girls] were psychologically under-
> mined by this differential treatment .... [However] an outcome of
> this pupil awareness of negative teacher evaluations of them was
> that black children refuse to present their real selves in school.
>
> (Mirza, 1992: 55)

Mirza also observed that the girls spent a lot of their time 'using strategies to avoid the effects of racist and negative teacher expectations'
(1992: 192). This resulted in the girls devoting less time to the activity of
learning. The Black Child Report (1999–2000) found that 22 per cent
of young black people in their study felt that they had experienced
racism from their teachers over the previous four weeks. A recent study
showed that 70 per cent of teacher training students have overtly racist attitudes (Jones, 1999). Another study found that only 30 per cent
of newly qualified teachers felt equipped to deal with diverse students
(Multiverse, 2004). In their interactions with teachers, black pupils
become disappointed and overburdened and 'learn helplessness', or
just lose interest in school (White and Cones, 1999).

Black people and members of other groups classified as numerical minorities may be subject to 'stereotype threat' or 'stereotype
vulnerability' (Steele and Aronson, 1995). This vulnerability refers to
the pressure experienced by a member of a stereotyped group in a performance situation where he or she is at risk of confirming a negative or
pejorative stereotype. For black pupils academic performance situations
increase concerns about confirming or being judged based on beliefs
regarding the intellectual abilities of their racial group. This impaired
performance is reflected in what Steele and Aronson (1995) describe as
the over prediction phenomenon. In these situations, even when African
Americans are academically capable (as reflected in aptitude scores that
are comparable to their European American peers) they demonstrate
lower academic performance. Steele and Aronson (1995) argue that
this lower performance may be due to processes associated with the
priming of racial stereotypes about academic performance. In a study
of college students in the US, Steele and Aronson (1998) showed that
having students identify their race before taking a test may cause worse
performance due to perceived 'stereotype threat', causing a 'disrup-
tive apprehension'. The race-primed black students felt apprehensive
because they equated identifying their race with feeling the need to
disprove stereotypes about their intelligence. By contrast, the scores of
race-primed white students did not significantly change in comparison
to white students who were not race-primed.

Not all teacher expectancy studies resulted in a finding consistent with the above studies (see, for example, Claiborn, 1969; Fleming and Anttonen, 1971; Foster, 1990). Foster, for example, argues that 'there is very little empirical support for the theory that teachers' negative racial views and low expectations are a major factor in explaining the relatively low educational attainment of Afro/Caribbean students' (Foster, 1992: 269).

Kunjufu maintains that 'research has shown that [teacher] expectations [are] the major factor in student achievement' (1985: 32). In a study of successful teachers of urban black students, Uhlenberg and Brown (2002) found that 'fundamental to their [teachers] beliefs about teaching was that all of the students could and must succeed. Black students seem to be more sensitive to their teacher's perception than their white classmates are' (Uhlenberg and Brown, 2002: 499). The authors conclude that 'teacher expectations could have a potentially significant influence on inner city black student performance' (2002: 500).

One additional statistic that seems to imply low expectations is the identification of black students for special services. Black children in US have been over-represented in special education classes (Boyd-Franklin *et al.*, 2001). This contrasts with the under-representation of black pupils in classes for the gifted (Boyd-Franklin *et al.*, 2001).

As noted above, research suggests that in Britain African-Caribbean students have been over-represented in special education provision (German, 2002; Majors, 2001). Black pupils are often labelled as behaviour problems or school failures at an early age (Boyd-Franklin *et al.*, 2001; Kunjufu, 1985). Such labeling often leads to special education placement and a higher risk for becoming a school dropout (Boyd-Franklin *et al.*, 2001).

African Caribbean boys are also four to six times more likely to be excluded from school than their white counterparts (Centre for Educational Research, 2003; Gillborn and Mirza, 2000). Majors (2001) argues that this finding could be an underestimate of the true figures. Black boys may be highly represented in 'informal' exclusions. The majority of black boys are unlikely to return to mainstream education once they have been excluded, thus being further disadvantaged. Britain has the highest rate of school exclusions in Europe (*Times Educational Supplement*, 19 January 2001). According to German (2002: 215) 'the fundamental reason for this lack of real progress is institutionalized racism based on unquestioned assumptions and unexamined practices. This racism includes a crippling combination of negative prejudice, destructive stereotyping and low expectations'. Research shows that stereotypes of black boys and girls persist. Their masculinity or femininity is interpreted by white teachers as 'sexualised' and 'aggressive' (Gillborn and Youdell, 2000). Bangladeshi and Pakistani youth are viewed as volatile, sexist and anti-authority (Alexander, 2000).

Implications of these findings for the placement of teachers in classrooms for work with black children are significant. In his book *Countering the Conspiracy to Destroy Black Boys*, Kunjufu (1986) states that he starts all his teacher workshops by declaring:

> You cannot teach a child who you do not love. You cannot teach a child who you do not respect. You cannot teach a child who you do not understand. You cannot teach a child if your 'political baggage', i.e. sexism and racism, is brought into the classroom.
>
> (Kunjufu, 1985: 32)

The black family and academic achievement

As pointed out earlier in Chapter 4, the majority of critiques and discussions of the black family have generally portrayed it as a social system that is disorganized, matriarchally dominated, and single-family directed (Boyd-Franklin *et al.*, 2001; Boyd-Franklin, 2003; Moynihan, 1965; Rainwater, 1970). This view of the black family has served as the basis for examining the issue of academic achievement. A consequence of this viewpoint has been the deficit-deficiency model of the black family as the explanatory paradigm (White, 1984, 2004) (see Chapter 4). In an article entitled 'Disadvantaging the disadvantaged: Bangladeshis and education in Tower Hamlets', Tomlinson presents evidence that 'dominant beliefs in family pathology still take precedence over analysis of the situation of disadvantaged groups in terms of structures and policies' (Tomlinson, 1992: 445).

Parekh (1983) has remarked on the 'fallacy of the single factor', the view that the black (African-Caribbean) family or culture was the most important factor in explaining the achievement gap. The earlier studies on educational achievement and the black child had a tendency to 'blame the victim' – by concentrating on the social background of pupils and ignoring the possible influences of the school. Some of the later studies have emphasized the role of the school. Tomlinson contends that:

> Out of the diverse explanations offered for minority pupils' performance, many of them concentrating on the supposed deficiencies of minority backgrounds, cultures, or languages, the school has

been particularly singled out as the most important agent for ensuring that minority pupils achieve well.

(Tomlinson, 1991: 137)

In the first major study on the effects of multi-racial schools, Smith and Tomlinson (1989) conclude that 'the school an ethnic minority child attends makes far more difference to his or her educational achievement than ethnic background' (Tomlinson, 1991: 137). However, Drew and Gray maintain that:

> To date we lack a study with a sufficient number of pupils and schools, covering a sufficient range of variables, with a nationally-representative sample, combining both qualitative and quantitative forms of data-gathering to answer the questions Swann posed.
>
> (Drew and Gray 1991: 171)

Cassen and Kingdon (2007: 3) found that 'disadvantaged students are likely to attend worse-performing schools. This can affect their outcomes adversely and does so particularly for minority ethnic students and students with Special educational needs'. According to the authors, 'anything which gives schools greater opportunities to select their pupils works to the detriment of the disadvantaged' Cassen and Kingdon (2007: 3).

An undermining aspect of black family research has been its insistence on comparing black families with white families. The underpinnings of such an approach assume that there is equality of opportunity and equivalency of life space between black and white families. It also implies that 'white' is the standard (White, 2004). Korchin argues that 'Still deeply ingrained is the assumption that the proper approach to the study of a minority people is to compare them to White' (Korchin, 1980: 263). This is the main criticism of research that interferes with arriving at more accurate and suitable explanations of the phenomena under study; this viewpoint is further underlined by Nobles (1978). This belief has, in respect of research on black families, led to a high-lighting of and preoccupation with the weaknesses of the family, with little or no focus on its strengths. As noted in Chapter 4, a strength that is well documented in the lives of black people is that of educational or achievement orientation (see Chapter 4) (Boyd-Franklin *et al.*, 2001, 2004; McAdoo, 2002). The 'salience of strong achievement orientation in black families is often unrecognized by whites who do not see this exhibited according to their own cultural expectations' (2004: 21).

Another criticism of black family research is that, for the most part, the family has been studied as if it were isolated from its environmental context. Any explanation of the black family, and its subsequent role and impact on academic achievement of its members, must acknowledge the fact that the family is embedded within a larger social system, that is, a system with reciprocal interactions and relationships that often do not enhance its best interest.

A number of studies (for example, Billingsley, 1968; Hill, 1972, 1999; Ladner, 1971; Nobles, 1974; Stack, 1974) have challenged the portrayal of the black family as pathological and disorganized and have attempted to explain the dynamics of the black family in a way that highlights its strengths. As discussed in Chapter 4, Hill (1972, 1999) presented strengths or factors that have helped black families to keep going under less than ideal circumstances. These included strong orientations to work, religion, achievement, strong kinship bonds, and role flexibility by family members. Hill states that: 'One of the unheralded strengths of blacks is the strong achievement orientation of low-income black families' (1972: 27). Black people have always valued education and have had strong achievement orientation (Boyd-Franklin *et al.*, 2001; McAdoo, 2002). Many view education as the way their children can have a better life. For poor parents, education is viewed as their children's chance for upward mobility (Billingsley, 1992; Hill, 1999). Black families 'place great value on education and knowledge as a way of counteracting the effects of oppression and discrimination. The desire for education is expressed in the long-standing institutions of Saturday schools located in black communities' (Graham, 2007: 84). In another study, Barn (2006: 58) found that 'black and Asian parents express higher education aspirations for their children' than white people.

There has always been a strong black educational movement. Black voluntary groups have set up their own schools (supplementary or Saturday schools) where basic skills as well as other aspects of the school curriculum were taught to black children (Majors, 2001; Mirza and Reay, 2000). The ethos is one of child-centred pedagogy and a shared inclusive curriculum, not often visible in 'mainstream' schools. Community schools such a these include those for Muslim and Jewish communities (Kempadoo and Abdelrazak, 2001).

Mirza points out that:

> When parental background *is* discussed with regard to black educational performance, it is nearly always done so in a negative light. The logical assumption is made that black children from low socio-

economic backgrounds must be influenced in the same way as their white counterparts, only worse (for example Swann, DES 1985).

(Mirza, 1992: 168)

Recent studies on the black family have continued to corroborate the work by Hill and other authors, by identifying the factors that help black family members in meeting their needs (Nobles, 1986). These studies have been successful in identifying the black family as a unit that helps to promote the academic achievement of black children, but they have not addressed the question of how achievement is supported and encouraged. Clark (1983) has attempted to answer this question in his study of why poor black children succeed or fail. He 'is one of the few researchers to offer insight into what he calls the "quality of life" in poor black homes' (Mirza, 1992: 168). Clark (1983) argues that family disposition (i.e. beliefs and values), as opposed to family composition (i.e. single-parent families or others), determines achievement orientation in children. In a study of young (15–19-year-old) black women attending two comprehensive schools in south London, Mirza found that 'black girls ... did seem to derive much of their determination for "getting on" from their parental orientation .... It was apparent that West Indian parents did encourage their daughters and were proud of their successes in many different ways' (Mirza, 1992: 176).

An extensive study by Clark (1983) of academic achievement of ten low-income black families with ten high school seniors (five high achievers and five low achievers) who were classified into one of four distinct family groups: two-parent families/one high-achieving senior; one-parent families/one high-achieving senior; two-parent families/one low-achieving senior; and one-parent families/one low-achieving senior, identified sixteen comparisons of the quality of success-producing patterns in the homes of high achievers and low achievers. The patterns for the high achievers were as follows:

1 there was frequent school contact initiated by the parents
2 the students had some stimulating and supportive teachers
3 parents were psychologically and emotionally calm with students
4 students were psychologically and emotionally calm with parents
5 parents were expected to play a major role in the children's schooling
6 parents expected their children to get post-secondary training
7 parents had explicit achievement-centred rules and norms
8 students showed long-term acceptance of norms as legitimate
9 parents established clear specific role boundaries and status structures with parents as dominant authority

10   siblings interacted as an organized subgroup
11   conflict between family members was infrequent
12   parents frequently engaged in deliberate achievement training
13   parents frequently engaged in implicit achievement-training activities
14   parents exercised firm, consistent monitoring and role enforcement
15   parents provided liberal nurturance and support
16   parents deferred to child's knowledge in intellectual matters.

These home patterns were the opposite for the low achievers. Clark asserts that his study 'demonstrates that specific qualities of family functioning are required to prepare children for competent school behaviour from kindergarten through high school' (Clark, 1983: 216).

Research on black families and academic achievement needs to redirect its agenda to the significant psychosocial patterns of family life that facilitate and maintain successful achievement. The research enterprise would do well to relinquish its preoccupation with the weaknesses of black families, and focus on the variables that make successful families function maximally. The results of various other studies (for example, Matthews-Juarez, 1982) strongly support the premise that successful academic achievement is a function of good parenting skills, positive parent involvement in the student's educative process, and other associated psychosocial variables. However, White (1984) contends that one cannot ignore a child's motivation to respond to the family's support and encouragement. He argues that, since there is little assurance of a payoff in the end, it does not make sense to black children to expend the time or effort to achieve. Thus, when a lack of payoff, limited visibility of successful blacks, and the realities of underemployment and unemployment are combined, it is not difficult to understand how these conditions alter the black child's perceptions to the extent of adversely influencing the pursuit of academic achievement (White, 1984; Parham *et al.*, 1999). Several studies (for example, Craft and Craft, 1983; Dove, 1974; Fuller, 1980; Tomlinson, 2005) have noted that black pupils in Britain show greater persistence in obtaining academic qualifications than their white counterparts. However, Fowler *et al.* have observed that 'increased education has less often led to increased pay-off for immigrants [black people]' (1977: 78). Tomlinson suggests that:

> Attitudes to school are closely linked to pupils' understanding of their situation in society generally, and although ... minority pupils and their parents do aspire to success in education and have positive attitudes towards staying on at school and moving into further and higher education (Fowler *et al.*, 1977; Gupta, 1977; Craft,

1980), there is also a realistic understanding of racial disadvantage and discrimination.

(Tomlinson, 1983: 123)

Lewis and Looney (1983), in their study of well-functioning working class black families, discuss the messages these families gave their children about how they can "make it" in spite of discrimination. Education is seen as the way out of poverty for African American/ black families, as it is for other ethnic groups. For some African American families who value education, the ability to translate this in terms of their children's schooling has not been accomplished. This is particularly true for some inner city black families who feel powerless to change their schools and who have been made to feel unwelcome in these institutions (Boyd-Frankiln, 1989; Boyd-Franklin *et al.*, 2001). Many African American parents find that it is very difficult for their children to perform consistent with the parents aspirations and goals for them (Hill, 1999; McAdoo, 2002). Boyd-Franklin (2003) observes that the 'largest number of referrals for therapy for African American children and adolescents are for school-related academic and behavioural problems. It is important for clinicians to understand the reasons for this discrepancy.'

Finally, Murray and Fairchild suggest that 'the solution to the comparatively poorer academic performances of Black American adolescents … should be aimed at the macro (i.e. systemic discrimination) and micro (i.e. teacher and student attitudes and behaviours) forces producing academic underachievement among Black adolescents' (Murray and Fairchild, 1989: 241). I believe that an understanding of both the micro and the macro forces is essential in understanding the underachievement of black children and adolescents in Britain.

Social work implications

The academic achievement of black children, generally speaking, has not been satisfactory. The most persistent conclusion of achievement research has been that of underachievement by black pupils in examination results. I have discussed the main factors affecting academic success.

Several challenges face social workers, school systems, the black community, and indeed the pupils themselves. The issues facing black children in schools need to be addressed. These include under-achievement, institutional racism, school exclusion and racial bullying in schools. The publication of the Stephen Lawrence Inquiry (Macpherson, 1999) heralded a brief but highly significant period when the issue of racism in public institutions was placed high on the political and media agenda. Although the police service was at the centre of the Lawrence inquiry itself, other public services (especially education) were also implicated in its findings.

A challenge within schools is to develop a healthy self-esteem among black pupils. Powell-Hopson and Hopson argue that 'there is a direct connection between [children's] self-esteem, their racial identity, and their academic achievement' (1990: 137). Social workers must help black children work through issues of identity development and find ways to enhance the black child's self-esteem. As the black child grows older, a knowledge of black history and black culture can strengthen his/her black identity. It is apparent that all children need to be educated about the positive contributions of black people in areas such as science, politics, business, athletics, art, literature, etc.

In their book on *Raising Black Children*, Comer and Pouissant (1992) suggest some ways that black parents can help their child develop a positive self-concept. They state that:

> As the child grows older, learning black history and experiencing black culture can strengthen his pride and broaden his sense of identity. Teaching a child strategies to deal with racism and the negative feelings about being black that racism incurs is very helpful .... With such preparation black children are able to maintain positive feelings about themselves when growing up in racist environments, whereas those without proper preparation often have low levels of self-esteem.
>
> (Comer and Pouissant, 1992: 16)

Powell (1982) (cited in Parham and White, 1999) put forward some suggestions for strengthening the self-concept of black children. These suggestions included: 'maximum participation by parents, teachers, [and social workers]; mores and values of the home reinforced in the immediate community and school; black culture and life styles reflected in the educational curriculum; academic achievement being encouraged regardless of social class' (Parham and White, 1999: 96). Graham notes that 'Culturally based epistemologies have received little attention in the development of an inclusive curriculum that reflects the multicultural nature of British society' (Graham, 2001: 66).

Social work models have tended to pathologize black families and encourage practitioners to perceive the families as being the 'problem'. Consequently, social work intervention focuses almost exclusively on clients' weaknesses, inabilities, and inadequacies. Social workers need to mobilize the strengths and competence in black families. Other challenges for social workers include resisting poor teacher expectations and stereotyping of black pupils.

However, 'the failure of central government to require a culturally relevant curriculum for all, and to make concerted efforts to train and appoint black teachers who would act as role models results in black young people feeling marginalized in a society which gives little positive recognition to diversity' (Barn, 2001: 40).

7 Black people and mental health issues

Introduction

This chapter is concerned with the Eurocentric and black perspectives which have sought to define black people's mental health problems. It describes the nature of the problems that black people face with regard to the psychiatric services. Central to examining the mental health status of blacks is the development of mental health definitions, classification, assessment methods, and treatment, from the black perspective. In this chapter I will discuss how a black perspective in psychology can inform and direct social workers and mental health practitioners in their work with black clients.

Deficiencies in the eurocentric perspective

The question one must ask is do psychological theories that originate in Euro-American, white middle-class-dominated clinical settings have relevance in working with black clients?

The 'albatross of racism and oppression has overshadowed thinking in Western-Eurocentric psychology and all of Social Science since its inception in the nineteenth century' (Jackson-Lowman, 2004: 599). As discussed in Chapter 1, a number of black psychologists (for example, White, 1972, 2004; Thomas, 1971; Nobles, 1976) have pointed out that traditional psychological theory does not deal adequately with the experience of blacks. Textbooks on abnormal psychology (for example, Davison and Neale, 2001) tend to ignore these issues. The writings of a number of authors (for example, White, 1972, 1999; 2004; Thomas, 1971; Nobles, 1976) are the basis for a theory of black psychology which more adequately addresses the issue of the uniqueness of the black experience and its relevance to the psychological functioning of black people.

What constitutes mental health for black people needs to be understood in the context of their own culture. Eurocentric standards of mental health are often inappropriate for black people, because they are based on the philosophies, values, and mores of Euro-American culture; variables used to develop normative standards of mental health. What constitutes sane or insane behaviour, mental health or mental illness, or normal or abnormal behaviour is, therefore, always in relation to a white normative standard. These standards are applied to black people by mental health workers who usually have little or no understanding of the black community's cultural requirements (Baughman, 1971; Kambon, 1998; White, 2004). Any diagnostic scheme dealing with blacks which fails to recognize the truth of black experiences and does not adequately provide for their inclusion in interpretative data is not only inadequate but profoundly unfair (Jackson-Lowman, 2004; Shannon, 1973).

Psychology is premised on the belief that the Western model is not only universal but is good. Throughout the history of Eurocentric psychology and psychiatry the diagnosis of personality functioning in black people has been objectionable. This is especially true of the diagnosis of personality disorder where early Eurocentric practice advanced diagnoses like drapetomania, in which escape behaviour by an enslaved African was considered a disease of the mind, and dysaesthesia Aethiopica, in which an African's resistance to enslavement was seen as a hebetude of mind (Thomas and Sillen, 1972). It was argued that 'freed slaves showed a much greater proneness to mental disorder because by nature the negro required a master' (Thomas and Sillen, 1972: 61). This kind of pernicious misrepresentation of black people's psychological functioning continued as Eurocentric psychology matured (see Guthrie, 1976, 2003), and has been immensely damaging to the health and welfare of blacks. Thus, similar to the dilemma regarding the Intelligence Quotient (discussed in Chapter 6), black people find their behaviour being judged against inappropriate standards and values, with any differences being interpreted as black psychopathology.

There has been relatively little written about the unique aspects of black mental health. Prior to the 1970s, the most widely cited books were Kardiner and Ovessey's *The Mark of Oppression* (1951; discussed in Chapter 5) and Grier and Cobbs' *Black Rage* (1968). Both works stressed the negative impact of racial oppression on the psychological development of black people. According to Kardiner and Ovessey, 'the Negro has no possible basis for a healthy self-esteem and every incentive for self-hatred' (1951: 297). Akbar (1991) considers that Kardiner and Ovessey's work makes an important contribution to the psychological literature on black people because:

> Oppression is an inhuman condition which stimulates unnatural behaviour ... [however] the over-riding problem with [their] book and the subsequent numerous related ones was the perspective of pathology accepted by these writers. All of the case histories presented suffer from some type of sexual and/or aggressive malady, not unlike any human being subjected to the Freudian microscope.
>
> (Akbar, 1991: 340)

Akbar also adds that 'the analysis of incompetent mental functioning is based on the norm and the context of the standards set by the middle class European American' (Akbar, 1981a: 341).

Many black people are increasingly challenging the concepts of normality and abnormality. They feel that their values and lifestyles are often seen by society as pathological, and thus are unfairly discriminated against by the mental health professionals. Some authors, for example, Akbar, argue that Western psychology's attempts to explain the problems of American blacks are inappropriate because: '1) [American Africans] are Africans (i.e. non-Western) in ... [their] basic dispositions; and 2) the quality of ... [their] environment (by the mere factor of oppression) is systematically different from the environment which Western writers use as the point of departure for understanding their condition' (Akbar, 1981a: 30).

Several authors have identified numerous deficiencies in much of the theoretical and empirical research on black people (see for example Billingsley, 1968; Guthrie, 2003; Jones and Korchin, 1982; Thomas and Sillen, 1972; Willie *et al.*, 1973, for detailed reviews). Some of the major concerns cited in the literature are:

1 diagnostic errors attributed to test bias (Williams *et al.*, 2004)
2 the lack of sufficient black psychiatrists and psychologists
3 the lack of understanding about black behaviour patterns from their own frame of reference
4 the lack of a general theory to outline the effects of racism on mental health
5 the lack of a general theory to describe normal and abnormal functioning in black communities
6 the application of majority-group-derived measures to blacks
7 a tendency to generalize to the larger black population on the basis of studies with small samples

8 a tendency to study the lowest income group and captive groups
9 a great emphasis on racial comparative paradigms
10 denial of the importance of intraracial comparative paradigms and the need for research on large, representative samples of blacks
11 a tendency to focus on pathology rather than strengths.

As a consequence, much of what is known about black mental health must be regarded with caution.

The major issues identified in the literature with regard to mental health and black people in Britain are: the over-representation of black people in mental institutions; the type of admission; diagnosis and the process of diagnosis (in particular the diagnosis of schizophrenia); and treatment.

In any discussion of incidence and prevalence of mental illness rates among blacks, we need to recognize that racism influences those factors that contribute to mental disorder, as well as those that affect the duration and severity of an illness. If one attempts to gain an overview of mental illness as it relates to black populations (both in this country and the United States), an examination of the literature will readily reveal that blacks are perceived to be more prone to psychological disorders than whites, and characteristically to have higher rates of mental illness. Thomas and Sillen argue that: 'investigators have made generalizations about epidemiology of black psychiatric disorders based on very little evidence ... and often these speculations were used to reinforce racist concepts' (1972: 215).

Although psychiatrists in Britain disagree about the incidence of mental illness among the black population, and about the reasons for it, there is some agreement among them that British-born African Caribbeans are more likely than whites to be:

diagnosed as suffering from schizophrenia and less likely to be diagnosed as suffering from depression (Harrison *et al.* 1988);

referred to hospital under compulsory procedures of the Mental Health Act 1983 (Cope 1989);

referred to psychiatric hospital with the involvement of police under Section 136 of the Mental Health Act (Rogers and Faulkner 1987), referred to hospital by a court under Section 37 of the Mental Health Act or be classified as a restricted patient under Section 41 (Browne 1990);

referred from prison to a special hospital or regional secure unit under Section 47 for remandees and Section 48 for convicted offenders (Cope and Ndegwa 1991);

treated with large doses of psychotropic medication (Littlewood and Cross 1980).

(Francis, 1991: 81–2)

The 'single most consistently reported finding from research into mental illness among ethnic minorities over three decades is the high rate of psychotic illness, schizophrenia in particular, in African Caribbeans' (Raleigh, 2000: 35). Evidence from the field of mental health also continues to show that African and Caribbean men are over-represented in mental health services and are mostly found at the harsher end of services (Raleigh, 2000; Fernando, 2002). Viewing young Caribbean men as dangerous can lead to inappropriate interventions, including their over-representation in the most secure forms of mental health institutions (Morgan *et al.*, 2005) and in the use of medication to control their behaviour (Gudjonsson *et al.*, 2004). African Caribbean people with mental health problems are more likely to receive medication as the primary form of treatment, are less likely to receive psychotherapy and are increasingly likely to attempt suicide (McKenzie *et al.*, 2001).

The 2006 census of inpatient services in England and Wales (Commission for Healthcare Audit and Inspection, 2007: 35) in relation to black and minority ethnic communities found that for African and Caribbean people:

Rates of admission to hospital were three times higher than average; referral rates from general practitioners were lower than average and rates of referral from the criminal justice system were higher than average; there was greater involvement of police in referrals; rates of detention under the Mental Health Act 1983 were between 19 and 38 per cent higher than average; there were higher rates of detention in medium and high secure wards; there were higher rates of detention in medium and high secure wards; there were higher rates of control and restraint.

The report urges 'statutory agencies, in partnership with others, to plan and commission services that will improve the pathways of care for black and minority ethnic groups' (Commission for Healthcare Audit and Inspection, 2007:35).

The situation for the Asian community is virtually the reverse, with Asians under-represented in many services (Beliappa, 1991; Bhugra and Cochrane, 2001; Fernando, 2002). This could be because the Asian community in the UK feels that the available resources in the mental health field are inappropriate to their needs. There is, however, considerable evidence that schizophrenia is diagnosed more frequently among people of Asian origin than might be expected (Bhugra and Cochrane, 2001; Cochrane, 1977; Carpenter and Brockington, 1980; Dean *et al.*, 1981; Hitch, 1981; Giggs, 1986). Another study found that the most common diagnosis among Asian patients in Waltham Forest was depression (Khan, 1983). Pinto (1970) and McGovern and Cope (1987) found an excess of compulsory admissions among Asian samples, but others (Hitch and Clegg, 1980; Shaikh, 1985) found no differences. Most of the studies indicate that African Caribbeans and Asians are more likely than whites to be diagnosed as suffering from schizophrenia, and to be admitted to psychiatric hospitals under compulsory admissions (Bhugra and Cochrane, 2001). There is also growing evidence that alcohol-related morbidity is high in some communities of Asian men, particularly Sikhs (Bhui *et al.*, 1993; Fernando, 2002). More recent studies have shown that 'young Asian women have higher attempted suicide (Bhugra *et al.*, 1999), although they are less likely to have a history of mental illness than white women attempting suicide. Social and family related factors are frequently cited as precipitators of self-harm in young Asian women' (Raleigh, 2000: 45).

Biased diagnostic instruments

One of the most well-known diagnostic approaches is the American system known as DSM-III (DSM is short for the *Diagnostic and Statistical Manual of Mental Disorder*, and III refers to the third edition, published in 1980). The most recent edition is DSM-IV. Traditional assessment frameworks such as the DSM-III-R (third edition revised) and DSM-IV use a European worldview and behaviour as the standard of normality. This results in increased rates of misdiagnosis among black people. Diagnostic labels used to classify mental disorders come from diagnostic nosologies (e.g. DSM-IV) or theoretical orientations that have not been normed or influenced by cultural standards that differ from those of white populations (Parham, 2002).

Loring and Powell (1988) found, in a sample of US psychiatrists, that diagnosis using DSM-III (American Psychiatric Association, 1980) was influenced by the 'race' (and sex) of case vignettes. Francis *et al.*

consider that 'nosological categories in psychiatry, derived from within a Eurocentric theory and largely based on observations in European settings, are deficient and misleading in categorising and describing the experience of non-European people' (1993: 142). Sashidaran endorses this view in his discussion on the misdiagnosis of schizophrenia. He states that 'systematic errors in psychiatric interpretations of black people's difficulties, symptoms, experiences or behaviour … come about because of the cultural and Eurocentric bias in the theoretical framework that clinicians routinely use for assessment and diagnosis' (Sashidaran, 1993: 112). In a report entitled 'Inside Outside' Sashidharan (2003) reports that 'Patients from all ethnic minority groups are more likely than white majority patients to be misunderstood and misdiagnosed'. This is a betrayal of our most vulnerable communities.

The use of 'objective' psychological inventories as indicators of maladjustment places black people at a disadvantage. The test instruments used on black people have been constructed and standardized according to white middle-class norms. The diagnostic tools used to define personality deviance, such as the projective methods of personality assessment, the Rorschach and the Thematic Apperception Test (mentioned in Chapter 1), are based on the accumulation of certain signs (inferred from verbal responses) in proper proportion to reflect normality. The projective method of personality assessment rests on the assumption that the more unstructured methods of assessment (those that present the individual with highly ambiguous or inherently meaningless stimuli) obtain a qualitatively richer yield of the unique aspects of the individual personality. Careful interpretation of the data presumably allows clinicians to make inferences about the deep rather than surface structure of personality: the individual's needs, fears, conflicts, and defensive mechanisms and other dynamic aspects of personality. Cultural differences are not acknowledged in the determination of deviance. Jones and Korchin state that:

> Until more is known about the influence of ethnic cultures on responses to the Rorschach, it is only reasonable that standard scoring categories be applied with caution. [Furthermore], inferences about the meaning of responses to projective techniques are particularly vulnerable to cultural bias.
>
> (Jones and Korchin, 1982: 22)

There is considerable American literature on the likelihood of racial bias intrinsic to the Minnesota Multiphasic Personality Inventory (MMPI and MMPI-2) – personality tests that are widely used in the US and Britain. One major shortcoming of the MMPI and MMPI-2 is the failure to recognize the extent to which culture may play a significant role in black people's expression of distress.

Numerous studies document that blacks receive more severe diagnoses and tend to score higher on the MMPI paranoia and schizophrenia scales than their white counterparts (Gynther, 1972). The results obtained by many researchers also 'suggest that, compared with whites, more black normals are likely to be falsely identified as deviant, and fewer black patients are likely to be incorrectly classified as normal' (Gynther and Green, 1980: 269). If a group of blacks were administered a personality test, and it was found that they were more suspicious than their white counterparts, what would this mean? Some psychologists have used such findings to label blacks as paranoid. In Britain, there is considerable evidence of an excess of paranoia among black people (Bhugra and Cochrane, 2001; Ineichen, 1984; Ndetei, 1986). This pathological interpretation of paranoia has been challenged by many black psychologists as being inaccurate. These authors argue that, in order to survive in a white racist society, black people have developed a highly functional survival mechanism to protect them against possible physical and psychological harm. The authors perceive this 'cultural paranoia' as adaptive and healthy, rather than dysfunctional and pathological. Thus, the personality test that reveals blacks as being suspicious, mistrustful, and 'paranoid' needs to be understood from a larger social-political perspective. Black people who have been victims of discrimination and oppression in a culture that is full of racism have good reason to be suspicious and mistrustful of white society. Recent writers have argued that black people have adopted various behaviours that have proven important for survival in a racist society. Therefore, a black person who is experiencing conflict, anger, or even rage may be skilful at appearing serene and composed. This tactic is a survival mechanism aimed at reducing one's vulnerability to harm and exploitation in a hostile environment.

Jones and Korchin maintain that:

> [E]thnic differences on measures of psychopathology like the MMPI are less likely due to differences in actual level of adjustment than to differences in the meaning of items from one group to another. This ... implies that a different set of validation studies must be established for minority subjects.
>
> (Jones and Korchin, 1982: 22)

A number of other authors – for example, Snowden and Todman – also affirm that 'the MMPI has never established its validity as a diagnostic or assessment instrument with blacks' (1982: 211).

Other possible causes of diagnosis

In the above section, I chose to highlight and criticize biased assessment techniques and measures because of their widespread use in the US and Britain. Some of the other factors that are likely to increase the likelihood of misdiagnosis among black people are: socio-cultural disparities between the clinician and patient and negative stereotypes of black people (Adebimpe, 1981; Snowden and Todman, 1982).

It is important to note that the vast majority of black people who have been labelled psychologically disturbed, mentally ill, or abnormal have been evaluated and labelled by white diagnosticians. The majority of decision makers at every stage of treatment, from the initial contact with patients to their ultimate discharge from treatment, are white. The influence of black professionals in the treatment of other blacks remains minimal in comparison to the size and strength of the white majority. A number of stereotypes operate in the encounter between black people and the welfare agencies of the state. African Caribbeans are stereotyped as aggressive, excitable, and defiant, and images of Asian people as meek, passive, and docile. Their analyses of these culturalist stereotypes suggest a 'pathologization of cultural differences'. Other prevalent stereotypes are that: Asians are not 'psychologically minded'; Asians somatize mental distress and present only physical symptoms; Asians 'look after their own' within their extended family networks (Lawrence, 1982).

We need to question the implicit Eurocentric bias in psychiatrists' diagnosis of mental illness. Mental health, more than any other health field, depends on communication for diagnosis and therapy (Bains, 2005). Attention must be paid not only to what a patient says and does, but also to the cultural context of the client's communication (Favazza and Oman, 1978). Some authors (for example, Padilla and Ruiz, 1975) have observed therapists of Anglo-American origin or training in the United States diagnosing numerous clients of a different ethnic group as schizophrenic. This diagnosis is based solely on the basis of the client's belief in supernatural phenomena, a belief that was generally unacceptable to the interviewing clinician. This example of misdiagnosis based on Eurocentric bias and nosology system cannot be considered unique. Another US study (Baskin *et al.*, 1981), using both black and white psychiatrists as diagnosticians, examined the influences of client-therapist differences on diagnosis. The results indicated that white psychiatrists were more likely than their black counterparts to diagnose black patients as schizophrenic. In fact, the black psychiatrists, who were assigned a total of 271 patients (141 black and 130 non-black), diagnosed only two patients (both nonblack) as schizophrenic, while white psychiatrists diagnosed 15 per cent of their total case load and 20 per cent of the blacks as schizophrenic. Baskin *et al.* (1981) concluded that diagnosis was not an objective assessment, but was in fact an assessment of observable behaviour compared to the cultural standards of the psychiatrist.

Doctors in Britain will have been trained 'to recognise a classical picture of disease which has arisen in European culture and has therefore been described in European terms. It is too often assumed that this is the normal pattern for other people from other lands' (Tewfik and Okasha, 1965: 603). Some black authors (for example, Thomas and Comer, 1973) have argued that indicators of positive mental health among black people – such as a willingness to challenge the conditions of racism, an awareness of society's hostility towards black people, and a strong identity with one's own culture – could be perceived negatively by a psychiatrist unfamiliar with the black norm. British psychiatrists are likely to misinterpret black people's expressions such as grief, distress, and anger as signs of schizophrenia (Fernando, 2003; Littlewood and Lipsedge, 1981a, 1997). Furthermore:

> British psychiatrists, trained in the conventional manner, fail to correctly recognize the true medical significance of black patients' symptoms because they lack an adequate knowledge of the black person's culture and how it influences the manifestation of mental illness.
>
> (Mercer, 1993: 21)

The lack of relevant knowledge of African-Caribbean history, belief systems, etc., and of the influence such a cultural background could have on the manifestations of psychological distress in African Caribbeans, has led to errors in diagnosis. Consequently, inappropriate use of such categories as schizophrenia is being made (Fernando, 2003; Littlewood and Lipsedge, 1981b, 1997). It therefore 'appears likely that the elevated rates of classical schizophrenia reported among the West Indian born are exaggerated' (Littlewood and Lipsedge, 1981b: 318). Adebimpe (1981) has also found that in the US black patients run a higher risk of being misdiagnosed as schizophrenics, whereas white patients showing identical behaviours are more likely to receive diagnoses of depression. It has been repeatedly stated in the Eurocentric literature that depression is rarely found among blacks in the US and Britain. Black people are viewed as having a primitive character structure, and as being too jovial to be depressed and too impoverished to experience objective loss (Adebimpe, 1981). However, symptoms of depression are more accurately perceived by white psychiatrists when the patient is white than when the patient is black (Hanson and Klerman, 1974). The psychiatric literature has also contrasted the specific character of depressions among blacks and whites. It is usually asserted that somatic complaints are likely to predominate in blacks, while feelings of guilt and suicidal trends are more evident in whites. The reported difference has been attributed to variations in family structure, child-rearing practices, and cultural norms.

Given that diagnostic differences exist between blacks and whites, and that larger percentages of blacks are assigned the more serious diagnoses, many social scientists assert that these differences reflect inaccurate psychiatric assessments and diagnoses and not 'true prevalence' of mental illness (Adebimpe, 1981, 1994; Carter, 1974; Gullattee, 1969). Psychiatric misdiagnosis is a serious problem, as diagnosis serves as the basis of treatment, referral and subsequent discharge (Baskin *et al.*, 1981). The relationship between type of diagnosis, type of treatment, and ethnicity of patient has been documented in the literature (Cox, 1977). For example, Cox compared the diagnoses and treatment modalities of black and white mental health clients. He found that blacks, in comparison with whites, were more often labelled schizophrenic and that individual, group, and family therapy were often provided to whites, while black clients tended to receive institutional care. Regardless of the psychiatric diagnosis, blacks in the US and Britain receive harsher treatment (e.g. drug therapy, seclusion, and restraint) than their white counterparts, because blacks are typically perceived as more violent than whites.

More recent reviews of the psychiatric literature continue to show that black people are often stereotyped as not being psychologically minded, and as lacking the psychological sophistication and motivation necessary for successful therapy. The over-representation of black people in British psychiatric hospitals is attributed 'either to "cultural" factors which quintessentially distinguish blacks from whites or to notions of black pathology' (Sashidaran, 1993: 111).

Although Eurocentric psychology is mature at 125 years of age in 2004, its diagnosis of mental disorder in black people remains detrimental in contemporary times. Myers and King (1980) reported statistics that showed a trend towards the disproportionate diagnosis of African Americans as having more severe and more antisocial conditions. Lewis *et al.* (1990) present evidence that, for psychiatrists, the factor of race will substantially alter their perception of patients and will influence the type and severity of diagnosis as well as the mode of treatment. According to Fernando (2002: 108), 'psychiatric diagnoses continues to carry racist undertones .... racism in Western culture continues to permeate the disciplines of psychology and psychiatry in research, theory and practice'.

Over the years, a number of crude diagnostic pseudo-categories such as 'West Indian psychosis' and 'Caribbean psychosis' have come into operation. These categories have not been coined as a result of theory, and there is no research to legitimize their practical use. Littlewood (1988) noted that the diagnosis of cannabis psychosis is applied more frequently in the African-Caribbean population despite the lack of convincing evidence supporting a major aetiological role for cannabis in severe psychosis (Onyango, 1986). It has been argued that mentally ill British African Caribbeans are treated more punitively and more likely to be 'labelled' with diagnoses of schizophrenia or cannabis psychosis because of racist attitudes among psychiatrists (Littlewood and Lipsedge, 1981b; 1997; Mercer, 1984; Cox, 1986; Littlewood, 1988, 1992). The reality of racism as a major force within psychiatric decision making and treatment, though often denied, is central to any understanding of black people's experience of psychiatry. Black people who come into contact with the mental health services are more likely to receive medication than 'talking therapies' such as psychotherapy or counselling. Asians are rarely referred to psychotherapy services (Campling, 1989; Ilahi, 1988). Sashidharan (2003) reported that 'mentally distressed black people are more likely to be locked away, that rates of compulsory admission are markedly higher and that black and minority patients are more likely than white people to be assessed as requiring greater degrees of supervision, control and security' (*Independent on Sunday*, 2003).

Although there is some concern in Britain about racism in psychiatry, this has not led to the adoption of any particular strategies to counteract it. However, 'the challenges to both psychiatry and psychology are increasing, particularly from users of psychiatric services and from organizations run by black and Asian people' (Fernando, 2002: 109). Black psychologists, social workers, and professionals in the mental health field have criticized the application of inappropriate norms to the assessment of black people's problems. Most black professionals have condemned things such as IQ tests, personality inventories, and other measures of psychological characteristics as inappropriate and destructive to black people's well-being. These tests are, however, extensively used in the US and Britain.

Black perspective in mental health

In this section I will discuss the development of a black perspective in the diagnosis of psychological disorders. Because of the tendency of psychiatrists operating within a Eurocentric frame-work to misinterpret the psychological functioning of black people, some researchers have identified the need to relate black behaviour only to black norms (e.g., Clark, 1965; Baughman, 1971; Barnes, 1972; Baldwin, 1981; Azibo, 1984; White, 2004). As noted above, concepts of mental health are an integral part of the values and belief systems of the culture in which they are based, and must therefore be viewed in relation to their cultural context.

In order to reduce diagnostic errors we need new definitions of mental health and illness which reflect a black perspective. Black social scientists (mainly in the USA) have attempted to define mental health from a black perspective. Parham and Helms (1985) examine the relationship between a black person's racial identity attitudes and his/her mentally healthy behaviour. Parham and Helms argue that the development of pro-black attitudes may be indicative of healthy psychological adjustment, whereas attitudes that denigrate one's self as a black person, while at the same time promoting wishes to be white, may be psychologically unhealthy (see Chapter 5).

Other researchers, for example, Pugh (1972), regarded black behaviours such as over-assimilation, the wish to be white, and identification with whites, as psychologically unhealthy defence mechanisms. Attitudes and behaviours such as colour denial (Myes and Yochelson, 1949) and dependence on white society for self-definition (Thomas, 1971) may act as a defence mechanism against anxiety; nevertheless, they are psychologically unhealthy. Pro-black attitudes and behaviours, as opposed to negative attitudes and behaviours related to being black, may be suggestive of healthy psychological functioning (Thomas, 1971; Baldwin, 1984; Nobles, 1986) (see Chapter 5).

Akbar (1981b) attempted to define mental health from a black (African) perspective. He proposes that, rather than classify African-American behaviour as mentally healthy or mentally ill, behaviour should be classified as ordered or disordered. According to Akbar, 'the definition of normality and abnormality is one of the most powerful indications of community power' (Akbar, 1981a: 35). Black people do themselves a disservice by letting white psychiatrists, psychologists, and social workers define the mentally disordered. 'Akbar's notions of mental disorders are ... predicated on the notion of opposition or alienation from one's self' (Nobles, 1986: 97). According to Akbar (1981a), these individuals have been socialized to be someone other than themselves and their lifestyles represent a rejection of their African dispositions. In contrast, behaviours that stimulate and uphold the survival of one's self and one's people are seen as psychologically ordered. Akbar put forward a classification system of disorders among African Americans that result from being an oppressed group. His classification system assumes that oppression is an unnatural and inhuman phenomenon that encourages unnatural human behaviour. Thus, abnormal functioning (i.e. disordered behaviour) can be the result of: an alien-self disorder; anti-self disorder; self-destructive disorder; and organic disorder. Akbar asserts that:

> The alien-self disorder represents that group of individuals who behave contrary to their nature and their survival. They are a group whose most prevalent activities represent a rejection of their natural dispositions. They have learned to act in contradiction to their own well-being and as a consequence they are alien from themselves.
>
> (Akbar, 1991: 343)

The anti-self disorder refers to those who, in addition to being social-ized to be other than themselves, express 'overt and covert hos-tility towards the groups of one's origin and thus one's self' (Akbar, 1991: 345). The self-destructive disorder represents individuals' 'self-defeating attempts to survive in a society which systematically frustrates normal efforts for natural human growth' (Akbar, 1991: 346). Akbar considers these individuals to be the most direct victims of oppression. Organic disorders refers to those conditions which, 'are the result of physiological, neurological or biochemical malfunction' (Akbar, 1991: 348). He stresses that all four disorders stem from 'a psychopathic society typified by oppression and racism', a situation which must be changed for blacks to 'realize the full power of their human potential' (Akbar, 1981b: 25).

As outlined by Akbar there are many similarities in the experiences of black people in America and black people in Britain (for example, oppression and racism). We need to develop a similar classification system in Britain.

As noted above, Eurocentric psychology has failed to address per-sonality disorder in blacks. In response to the inadequacy of the DSM-III-R for the diagnosis of disorder in African Americans, Azibo (1989) developed a nosology for the assessment of personality disorders in blacks. The Azibo nosology (a nosology is an organized system for diagnosing diseases, disorders, or pathologies, as opposed to their simple listing) is 'a diagnostic system of ordered and disordered African (Black) personality functioning ... [that] systematizes 18 of the disorders of the African personality (a) with one another and (b) with the nosological system prevalent in Euro-American psychology (DSM-III)' (Azibo, 1989: 173). Hence, disorders that are specific to the African personality are found in the Azibo and not the DSM-III-R nosology. The Azibo nosology describes the 'systematic unfolding of disorder in the African personality'. It includes the disorders described by Akbar (1981b) and Thomas (1971). The nosology is linked to an Africentric perception of ordered or normal behaviour. Thus, 'correct orientation is described as genetic Blackness plus psychological Blackness ... [which means] conscious manifestation of African-centered psychological and behavioral functioning in genetically Black persons' (Azibo, 1989: 182). Misorientation is described as genetic blackness minus psychological blackness (Azibo, 1989). It is a psychological state in which an African operates 'without an African-*centered* belief system ... [s/he] proceeds with a cognitive definitional system that is non-Black ... [and] depleted of concepts of psychological Blackness and ... composed of alien (i.e., non-African) concepts [like] psychological Europeanism' (Azibo, 1989: 184–5).

Another concept proposed by Azibo (1989) is mentacide, which 'render[s] the African's psyche void of any pro-Black orientations to life ... simultaneously [there is] an instilling of (a) a pro-European orientation that commands ... acceptance and admiration of and allegiance to White persons and White-dominated society ... and (b) the relative disparagement of all things African' (Azibo, 1989: 186). It can be seen that mentacide produces misorientation. Azibo gives an example of a black female diagnosed with Panic Disorder. Panic attacks occurred when she was confronted with her own blackness. Treatment included helping the client to discuss and identify who she was, and address the issues of race. Similar issues and problems are apparent in Britain (for example, Maxime's (1997) work with black children in care; and Banks' (2002) direct 'racial' identity work).

It can be seen that Eurocentric methods of diagnosis (for example, DSM-III-R) hide the true nature of black personality disorganization, whereas the Azibo nosology unmasks it. In the case cited above, for example, the client's real condition was hidden by the (Eurocentric) DSM-III-R Panic Disorder diagnosis but was revealed by the Azibo nosology. Intervention proceeding from an Azibo nosology diagnosis is aimed at removing the personality disorders and producing what Azibo refers to as correct orientation/psychological blackness.

Personality theories of black people (African Americans), especially those articulated by Nobles (1986, 2004), Akbar (1981a, 2004), Baldwin (1984), Azibo (1983, 1987), and Parham and Helms (1985), stress the necessity of achieving congruence between the 'self' one wishes to become, and one's true (black) make-up if one is to be a fully functioning and well-adjusted individual. If there is an aspect or factor of personality that does not fit well with, function well with, or contribute constructively to the overall personality organization, then the efficient functioning of the personality is decreased or perhaps even seriously disrupted. Thus, attitudes and behaviours that devalue blackness, or that over-assimilate white cultural values, can be seen as representing degrees of incongruence between a black person's real self and idealized self because they violate the natural order of that person's black make-up.

Treatment issues for black people

Research continues to show lower rates of mental health service utilization by minorities in the US and the UK (Spencer and Chen 2004; Rabiee and Smith, 2007; Bhui 2002). There is still evidence of both over-exposure to acute services and the powers of compulsion, and simultaneously also of low utilization, restricted access, poor case detection, and inadequate referral (Rabiee and Smith, 2007). In Britain, as in the US, hospitalized black patients, compared with white patients, are more likely to be 'treated' with seclusion or other repressive conditions of 'care'– and the racist stereotype of 'black violence' is the basic reason for this (Fernando, 2002: 122). Rabiee and Smith (2007) found that African and Caribbean service users in Birmingham, on the whole, have negative perceptions of mainstream mental health services. In his report, 'Inside Outside', Sashidharan's (2003) concluded that 'mental health services [in Britain] were institutionally racist, that the whole issue of ethnicity within mental health services had become marginalised or even ignored and that these problems were getting worse'.

We must question the validity and usefulness of white-originated theories in the treatment of the mental health problems of black people. Many black psychologists argue that traditional psychological theories do not adequately take into account the unique characteristics of the black experience nor the importance of the historical/cultural aspect of black behaviour. Therefore, traditional psychological theories as applied to therapy/treatment have little or no utility in dealing with the mental health problems of blacks and other minorities.

The assumption that psychological theories are applicable to all groups of people, regardless of ethnic or cultural differences, has not been adequately evaluated or assessed. However, when the treatments evolving from these theories do not help the patient, the conclusion generally reached is that the patient lacks those qualities necessary for successful therapy. It is possible that the theory may not be applicable across different cultural or ethnic groups (Bhugra *et al.*, 1999); or the psychiatrist may have biases or prejudices that make it difficult for him/her to provide successful treatment.

As noted above, in Britain and the United States black patients are less likely than whites to receive psychotherapy but are more likely to receive physical treatment (Thomas and Sillen, 1972; Kaye and Lingiah, 2000; Littlewood and Cross, 1980). Blacks are often stereotyped in the psychiatric literature as not being psychologically minded, as culturally deficient, and as lacking the psychological sophistication and motivation to benefit from psychotherapy. Such ideas influence the criteria for patient acceptance, availability of facilities, form and length of therapy, nature of the patient-therapist relationship, therapeutic goals, and judgement of outcome.

The concentration of black patients in secure settings, where drugs and physical restraint are used as the main therapeutic tools, has led to the under-use of counselling, psychotherapy, and group work in these patients. This reflects a form of the classical racist-scientific view that black people are incapable of experiencing depression and that their under-developed linguistic and intellectual faculties render them unsuitable for psychotherapeutic treatment. Psychotherapy is denied to black patients because psychiatrists 'regard black patients as incapable of verbal self-expression of emotional difficulties' (Littlewood and Cross, 1980: 200).

Some of the reasons which have been put forward by professionals for the low referral of Asians to psychotherapy are:

- lack of confidence in the effectiveness of psychotherapy amongst general practitioners and other referring agents
- the perception of psychotherapy as a treatment for the 'privileged white middle-classes'
- the perception of Asians as lacking the capacity for psychological insight
- the perception of Asians as accepting that personal problems are external and beyond the individual's capacity to change
- the perception of Asians as thinking only in bodily (somatic) or spiritual terms
- lack of psychotherapists from the Asian community
- lack of psychotherapists who speak Asian languages

• cultural and/or language barriers in the initial stages of assessment.
(Webb-Johnson, 1991: 13–14)

These perceptions may be held by Asian as well as white professionals. Ilahi (1988) found that Asian doctors were reluctant to refer their Asian clients for psychotherapy (also see Bhui *et al.*, 2003).

If we examine the psychological literature, we find that stereotypes of typical white (mainly middle-class) clients match those characteristics (intelligent, motivated, verbal, attractive, articulate, personable, trusting, disclosive) that are most highly valued by therapists in ideal client populations. The question we therefore need to ask is: 'What is the degree of congruence between characteristics most highly valued in clients and those stereotypically associated with black groups?' Stereotypic attitudes of black clients conflict with the 'ideal client' characteristics. If black patients continue to be characterized as being less verbal, impulse-ridden, more concrete than abstract in thought, and having difficulty dealing with intrapsychic material, therapists may be encouraged to adopt more action-oriented, compared with insight-oriented, therapeutic strategies when working with black patients (Smith, 1977). However, evidence from organizations in Britain (for example, Nafsiyat Intercultural Therapy Centre which are providing psychotherapy to members of the Asian community) shows that Asians are able to benefit from this kind of therapy (Kareem *et al.*, 1999).

A psychotherapist's identification with white middle-class values is of great significance for the outcome of psychotherapy. This identification can affect the psychotherapist's feelings and attitudes about black behaviour (Bloch, 1968). Responses which seem unusual, inappropriate, or even pathological to the therapist might be quite consistent with the values of the patient's culture. A client's behaviour may not only reflect his cultural background but also the client's response to the racial feelings of the psychotherapist (Bloch, 1968). Consequently, it is not only necessary for a psychotherapist to understand a client's culture before he can be sure that the client is behaving inappropriately; it is also necessary for the psychotherapist to be aware of whether or not he is unconsciously communicating negative messages to the client. For example, as indicated above, it is common for black patients to be labelled as paranoid or at least hypersensitive to insults and other racial issues (Bloch, 1968; Fernando, 2002). The patient's expression of these feelings is often dismissed as defensive by the therapist, thus negating the validity of the client's perceptual world.

Littlewood and Lipsedge (1981a, 1997) and Fernando (2002) point to ethnocentrism operating within the psychiatric encounter with the black person. Black experiences are generally seen and analysed from the 'white middle-class perspective'. When black experiences are discussed, the focus tends to be on pathological lifestyles and/or maintenance of false stereotypes. Often stereotypes about black people are carried over into the therapy situation. It is often 'naively' assumed that 'professionals' have miraculously 'cleansed' themselves of racial and class biases. Therapists have the same cultural stereotypes, fears, and concerns about individuals of different races as the rest of the population. Some of the variables that interfere with the relationship between the black client and white therapist are:

> (1) the inability of white psychotherapists to comprehend the social, economic, and cultural customs of blacks; (2) lack of emphasis or awareness of the therapists' own feelings regarding race and class; (3) minimal scientific research on the particulars of black and minority behaviours; (4) utilization of theoretical constructs designed by and for whites to treat black patients; and (5) clinical training that is culturally deficient in that it does not communicate a black or minority mental-health perspective.
>
> (Smith *et al.*, 1978: 148)

In addition to an understanding of the black community and everyday black life, white therapists need to take a close look at their feelings relative to race (Bloch, 1968; Sue, 2006). The negative racial attitudes held by the white therapist may destroy the entire therapy process from the time the client comes in the door until the client is released. These attitudes have serious consequences for the black client as the psychotherapist, unaware of the effects of racial myths on his/her thinking, continues to misinterpret, mislabel, and misadvise. Various stereotypes about blacks seem to persist even when psychotherapists view the myths as untrue. Myths about aggressiveness and sexuality are particularly common. Consequently, black clients can arouse anxieties in the therapist. Although these anxieties may be too vaguely defined to be recognized by the therapist, they can, nevertheless, have a profound influence on his/her behaviour during a therapy session. Such anxiety can result in distorted perceptions of the black client's behaviour, in mishandling or overemphasis of the importance of certain client feelings and/or behaviours, and in neglect of areas of exploration which might have been fruitful.

Much of the blame for the perpetuation of racial myths and stereotypes in the mental health field is attributable to the vast psychological and psychiatric literature which psychotherapists study. Training in traditional institutions adversely affects the functioning of psychotherapists with black clients (Banks *et al.*, 1967). As discussed in Chapter 1, the 'scientific' literature concerning blacks has great potential for reinforcing racial stereotypes (Gardner, 1971; Fairchild, 1991). Stereotypes regarding the inferiority of blacks occur frequently in the literature (Thomas and Sillen, 1972), although genetic explanations have often been replaced by psychodynamic explanations (Gardner, 1971). Both Gardner (1971) and Thomas and Sillen (1972) provide excellent examples of the role of the literature in keeping the myths of race in the forefront of psychotherapeutic thinking.

Black perspective in therapy

> European models of counselling are not devised to take account of ethnic minority experiences and culturally different life experiences. The models need to be changed when dealing with ethnic minorities.
>
> (African-Caribbean mental health worker)

Increasingly, black theoreticians have questioned the application of traditional treatment approaches to black populations, citing as evidence the lack of congruence of these practices with the black experience, lifestyle, and culture (Akbar, 1977; Banks, 1972; Nobles, 1972; Vontress, 1971). As Eurocentric theories of mental illness dominate the psychological and psychiatric literature, most psychological intervention models (for example, Carl Rogers' client-centred or nondirective therapy and Freud's psychoanalysis) are of questionable value in providing maximal treatment benefits to black clients. Commenting on these matters, Jackson responds that the 'do-it-yourself aspect of the nondirective approach [Carl Rogers' therapy] is seen as threatening to the client and may result in the client's withdrawal' (Jackson, 1976: 297). He also views psychoanalysis to be unsuitable in the treatment of black clients (see Jackson, 1976). However, Maultsby (1982) considers behaviour therapy to be 'culture-free' and thus minimally biased against blacks. He concludes that in the US the most effective techniques for blacks are those of classical behaviour therapy, cognitive behaviour therapy, and rational behaviour therapy.

To counteract the negative view of black people, the black perspective was developed. American research on the black perspective in mental health is more advanced than in Britain and offers guidelines on how cross-racial therapy can respond to the needs of black clients in Britain. This perspective gives 'new interpretations of black behaviour and posits new images based upon strengths to supplant the old images based upon weakness' (Jackson, 1976: 301).

In relation to the therapeutic practices, it should be borne in mind that it is not simply a case of replacing, say, physical psychiatric treatment (drugs, ECT, restraint) with a Western psychotherapy whose concepts (such as the Oedipus complex, transference, and the relation between consciousness and the unconscious) may be thoroughly Eurocentric. It is necessary to develop techniques and approaches which are based upon black culture (Jackson, 1976). Azibo (1989) urges practitioners in the US to use the Azibo nosology and stresses the importance of developing Africentric psychotherapies that are directed to bringing about the personality state of correct orientation. Some work has been done in this area (see Myers, 1988, for a detailed description).

In Britain, a body of critical work has been emerging (for example, Dalal, 1988; Fernando, 2002; Kareem, 1988; Kareem and Littlewood, 1999). Kareem argues that 'recognition of cultural diversity forms a very important part of intercultural therapy' (Kareem, 1993: 152). He also notes that 'racism is ... [an] important dimension in inter-cultural therapy' (Kareem, 1993: 153). He suggests that black people do not refer themselves to traditional therapy centres because 'they pick up a message that "black people are like shit" and white people like milk ... and from this they conclude that they would not be fully accepted' (Kareem, 1988: 8). Kareem describes inter-cultural therapy as:

> A form of dynamic psychotherapy that takes into account the whole being of the patient – not only the individual concepts and constructs as presented to the therapist, but also the patient's communal life experience in the world – both past and present. The very fact of being from another culture involves both conscious and unconscious assumptions both in the patient and in the therapist ... for the successful outcome of therapy, it is essential to address these conscious and unconscious assumptions from the beginning .... So this means that when we are treating patients from black and ethnic minority groups we have to take up the issues of their real life experience of racism.
>
> (Kareem, 1988: 7)

Adams (1970) views racism, conscious or unconscious, as a factor that causes negative countertransference reactions, which interferes with successful psychotherapy. He therefore recommends that therapists themselves deal with this negative countertransference by undergoing personal psychotherapy. Therapists and social workers must also be aware that due to psychology's and psychiatry's negative perception and treatment of black people in the past, black people can have an understandable distrust of mental health professionals (Maultsby, 1982; McKenzie, 2003). In a recent study of African Caribbean interactions with mental health services, Mclean, Campbell and Cornish (2003) found that the African Caribbeans in their sample 'asserted that experience and expectation of racist mis-treatment by mental health services were key factors discouraging early accessing of mental health services, and thereby perpetuating mental health inequalities' (2003: 657). It is important to note that 'the experience of racism and racial discrimination is likely to have a bearing on the health status of all ethnic groups .... racial discrimination is a facet of the lives of all Britain's minorities' (Ali and Atkin, 2004: 67).

Black perspective in therapy: confronting denial of black identity

The body of theoretical knowledge on black psychology and mental health focuses on the concept of black identity formation, and the possibility that blacks go through a series of stages in their efforts to establish stable personalities (see Chapter 5). This concept of stages in black identity formation has led to the emergence of a body of empirical evidence which suggests that variation in black attitudes toward racial identity may have an effect on counselling process and outcome (Helms, 1986; Parham and Helms, 1981; see discussion below).

In psychotherapy with a black patient the issue of race must always be addressed. To deny the significance of the race of a black person as an important part of identity is to deny an important and overriding aspect of his/her being. The therapist must be comfortable in dealing with racial material and feelings; knowledgeable about and sensitive to the patient's customs and culture; and skilful in helping the patient to uncover and work through this material for the therapy to be successful (Ramseur, 2004). In treatment, denial of black identity may be exhibited by the patient or by the therapist. When the patient is unable to see him/herself and situations affecting him in the context of the identity, role, and circumstances of blacks in this society, he/she is denying his/her black identity. The denial requires a rejection of a significant part of self, and hence is an unhealthy attempt at adjustment. In treatment, the therapist helps the patient in recognizing the denial of his/her identity by helping him/her question and confront his/her perceptions and his/her use of denial. The therapist must assist the patient in uncovering, tolerating, and examining the fears, etc., underlying this defence. As the reality is seen, the client works through and resolves the conflicts and issues involved, and more appropriate mechanisms for coping are developed. With this comes the incorporation of a healthy black identity. When the therapist denies the significance of the patient's black identity, he/she has not resolved his/her own racism. This is usually apparent when the therapist sees the patient as 'not as a black, but just like everyone else'. This phenomenon of 'hallucinatory whitening' is a denial of the individual's black identity (Jones and Jones, 1970). In such cases, for the white therapist to see and relate to the black patient as a black person threatens the therapist's unresolved repressed racial conflicts. Thomas and Sillen (1974) pointed out that, for some therapists, it is easier and more comfortable to deny that racial differences exist and to see problems only in class or economic terms. Such a belief is (unfounded) and thus counterproductive, leading to what Thomas and Sillen (1974) have referred to as 'the illusion of colour blindness'. This phrase refers to the tendency on the part of many members of the mental health field to deny the impact of colour differences in therapy. As Thomas and Sillen explain, '"colour blindness" is no virtue if it means denial of differences in experience, culture, and psychology of black Americans and other Americans. These differences are not genetic, nor do they represent a hierarchy of "superior" and "inferior" qualities, but to ignore the formative influence of substantial differences in history and social existence is a monumental error' (Thomas and Sillen, 1974: 58). Block (1980) cautions service providers about being influenced by, and promoting the illusion of, colour blindness (e.g., 'I don't view you as a black person, I see you as a human being') (also see Dominelli, 1997).

Some psychotherapists are apt to make comments such as 'I treat them all alike'; 'when I look at you I don't see a colour, I see a person – a human being'. When the issue of colour is ignored by the therapist, a very important aspect of the client's reality is being ignored. The psychotherapist who considers himself/herself to be colour-blind can be just as harmful to black clients as an overt bigot. 'Colour-blind' psychotherapists are ill-equipped to deal with black clients because they have chosen to pretend that a significant feature of the client's life is unimportant. Bloch states that '… it is not likely that the white psychotherapist can escape all the negative connotations that the colour black symbolizes in western society' (Bloch, 1968: 279).

Racial identity states and the therapeutic relationship

The therapeutic relationship between the therapist and the client is a vital and necessary part of the therapeutic process (Highlen and Hill,

1984). Parham (1989) asserts that recognizing the within-group variability among black clients may assist a therapist in understanding how the racial identity attitudes of a client (discussed in Chapter 5) may influence his/her ability to establish a workable relationship with that client. Thus, white therapists who begin treatment with a black person possessing pro-white and anti-black attitudes (pre-encounter stage) will have little difficulty in establishing rapport with the black client. If the client is more immersed in his or her identity (immersion-emersion stage), he or she could have difficulty in establishing a relationship with the white therapist (Parham and Helms, 1985). The authors point out that positive therapeutic work can result if the 'client's perceptions of the therapist are worked through in the initial stages of therapy' (Parham and Helms, 1981: 256).

Due to the importance of trust, rapport, and communication in the therapy situation, it would be reasonable to assume that a black therapist would be more effective with black clients. Terrell and Terrell (1984) found that black clients high in cultural mistrust who were seen by white therapists for their initial visits to a community mental health center were less likely to return than blacks high in mistrust seen by black therapists. Black clients with severe disturbance who are also high in cultural mistrust prefer black clinicians, although they also believe that white clinicians are better trained (Whaley, 2001).

A number of studies have shown that black clients tend to prefer black counsellors and therapists (Heffernon and Bruehl, 1971; Gardner, 1971; Harrison, 1977). Other studies have demonstrated that black clients tend to have a more positive relationship (as well as outcome) when the therapist is black (Griffith, 1977). The idea which many black people hold – that 'you cannot disclose certain things to white professionals' (Channel 4, 1987) – emanates from a belief that their own values and ethics are diametrically opposed to those of professional social work or psychiatry (also see Fernando, 2002).

However, black therapists will also have to deal with their own feelings and attitudes towards blackness, as well as with those of their clients. If a black therapist is matched with a client with strong pre-encounter attitudes, the client might believe that the black therapist is less qualified than a white counterpart, and therefore less capable of providing effective treatment. As the number of black professionals is limited, many white professionals will be working with black clients. At Nafsiyat, Kareem points out, their therapists come from 'a variety of colours, races and cultures, from both sexes, and [they] do not necessarily match the patient with a therapist from the same cultural group' (Kareem, 1988:8). He adds that clients were more likely to request that the therapist be of a particular sex than a particular race or colour (Kareem and Littlewood, 1999).

In order to increase effectiveness with black clients, both black and non-black therapists and social workers need to be aware of the following issues: the impact of oppression on the lives of black people; black psychological perspectives as a source of strength; and racial identity states (White, 1984; 2004).

White racial identity development

Helms's (1984) five stage model of white racial identity was discussed in Chapter 4.

Helms's (1984) interactional model attempts to provide a framework that guides professionals (for example, social workers, mental health workers) in their effort to understand how 'race' and racial identity influences the counseling process and therapeutic relationship. Her framework considers within-group variation in interracial dyads through the use of the racial identity construct. Helms outlines the interactional dynamics that may occur in dyads as a result of the various combinations of racial identity attitudes held by the participants. Helms also extended racial identity theory to the group process (see Chapter 4).

Helms's original rationale for offering a framework was to enable counselors to diagnose tensions in the environment, and to intervene to resolve them in a manner compatible with the racial identity dynamics of the participants. Originally, 'environment' referred to dyadic counseling or psychotherapy relationships (Helms, 1984). Subsequently, the concept of environmental context was extended to refer to other dyadic interactions in which 'the participants differ in social power and/or status due to role expectations' (Helms, 1990: 177).

Helms's (1984) interaction theory, which builds on her racial identity theory, proposes that a person's stage of racial identity, rather than racial group membership per se, determines the quality of the communication process. Helms argues that different combinations of stages should result in different styles of communication. According to Helms (1984, 1990) there are four communication patterns; parallel, crossed, progressive and regressive (discussed in Chapter 4 in relation to the group process). In a parallel relationship a social worker and client share the same stages of identity. Parallel relationships are perhaps 'the least contentious of dyadic interactions because [the social worker and client] share a racial worldview' (Helms, 1990: 180). For example, a parallel relationship is formed when the black client is at the pre-encounter stage and the social worker is at the contact stage;

or when the black client predominantly exhibits encounter attitudes and the white professional is at the disintegration stage. In a crossed relationship, the worldviews of the client and the social worker are totally opposite. Helms (1990: 181) argues that these individuals will have 'difficulty in communicating with each other because they do not share any part of a common frame of reference where the racial parts of themselves are concerned'. A progressive relationship exists when the social worker's racial identity is at least one level above the client's. A regressive relationship exists when the client's racial identity status is at least one level more advanced than the worker's.

The following illustrates an example of a form of regressive dyadic interaction that can occur in a social work interview with a black adolescent. The black adolescent may want to talk about racism in his/her school and the attitudes of teachers to black students. The social worker, however, may insist that such issues should not be important to the young person. The black adolescent can feel disrespected and devalued in this situation. The social worker risks miscommunication if he or she cannot allow the client to develop the racial aspects of self.

Implications for social work

What implications does a black perspective in the assessment, diagnosis, and treatment of mental disorders have for social workers who work with black clients? Clarke *et al.* (1993) point out that:

> Historically and currently, psychiatry occupies the dominant role within mental health provision, and social work has been strongly influenced by mainstream psychiatric thinking. Social workers, alongside psychiatrists, exercise power over users of services. This may be at the everyday level of offering or withholding particular forms of help, or the exercise of legal powers in over-riding someone's objections to hospital admission.
>
> (Clarke *et al.*, 1993: 172)

In order to work effectively with black clients, social workers need to familiarize themselves with the black perspective in the assessment, diagnosis, and treatment of mental disorders. This perspective represents an important contribution towards social work knowledge. In a study of approved social workers' assessment of black people, Mani Shah (1990) found that the social workers were operating within a Eurocentric model of care. For example, some social workers were adopting a colour-blind approach – 'I treat everybody the same';

'There is no difference between white or black clients – if they are ill they are ill'.

It is important that the social worker disentangles him- or herself from implicit racial and cultural stereotypes. For instance, the assumption that black people are not articulate and cannot constructively engage in therapeutic encounters involving active verbalization needs to be challenged by social workers. If left unchallenged, negative stereotypical images about the black client's family organization, choice of partners, and child-rearing practices can become the basis for everyday knowledge for the social worker. In working with black people it is important for the social worker not to attribute all the client's problems to some 'cultural' peculiarity on the one hand, while, on the other, neglecting cultural variability with the aim of treating everyone the same. Dominelli notes that social workers adopt various strategies, one of which is the colour-blind approach in order to 'deny, ignore and minimize the presence of racism in their own institutions, culture and personal behaviour' (Dominelli, 1992: 166–7).

Social workers and psychotherapists should be provided with frequent opportunities to examine their feelings about blackness, and to evaluate the relevance to black people of psychotherapeutic theories, research, and techniques. Without a conscious awareness of attitudes and anxieties that may be stimulated by the presence of a black client, the effectiveness of a social worker's interventions will be seriously diminished. Few social workers attempt to become aware of their racial feelings. It seems more common for social workers and mental health workers to assume that such feelings have been replaced either by a professional approach to all patients or by a conviction that, somehow, they are different from other white people when dealing with the issue of race. Social workers and psychotherapists must be aware that merely studying black history or reading black books is no guarantee that the white therapist will be able to treat black people more effectively. The process of eliminating one's racial bias is much more difficult and involves an in-depth analysis of oneself and of a society that has fostered racism and oppression – it is a long-term process.

Racial identity model (discussed in Chapter 5) 'has been theorized to significantly influence cross-racial counseling relationships .... [it] has recently been identified as particularly important to understanding multicultural counseling processes and cross-cultural relationship development' (Burkard *et al.*, 2003: 226). Social workers need to 'understand that the level of White racial identity development in an interracial encounter ... affects the process and outcome of an interracial relationship (including social work practice)' (Sue, 2006: 127). Tuckwell (2002) notes that white therapists need to examine the impact of white racial identity on their practice. Some of the areas highlighted by Tuckwell (2002: 6) include: 'raising their [the therapist's] awareness of the ways in which their own racial identity influences their therapeutic practice; recognizing how their own biases, beliefs and assumptions impact on their work with clients; identifying and exploring their emotional reactions to racially different clients'.

Social workers need to have an understanding of white and black identity development and its effects on interracial counselling. For example, pro-black and anti-white attitudes of a black client could be interpreted by the social worker as a stage in black identity development and not as a personalized attack. It is important to recognize the dangers in this situation of the insight obtained by the use of identity theory becoming corrupted into lazy psychological reductionism. The social worker's acknowledgement of the client's racial identity attitudes must not replace their sensitivity to and knowledge of the client's experience of exclusion and discrimination on the grounds of 'race'.

As noted above, in the pre-encounter stage the black client is most likely to prefer a white worker over a black worker. Consequently, a white social worker may have little difficulty breaking down the social distance and establishing a working alliance between him or herself and the client where ethnicity is concerned. The black client at this stage believes that white social workers are more competent and capable than black workers. If a black social worker is matched with a client with strong pre-encounter attitudes, the client might believe that the black worker is less qualified than a white counterpart and therefore less capable of providing effective care. Black social workers may encounter negative reactions, resistance or open hostility. Maxime (1997: 105) notes that 'many black social workers have experienced comments such as "I don't want a black social worker", "don't come near me", or verbal and sometimes physical abuse'. Maxime (1993) (a black clinical psychologist) encountered negative reactions when she attempted to do clinical work with a black girl at the pre-encounter stage. In this stage, the child usually makes a request for a white psychologist/ therapist' (Maxime, 1993: 106). Parham and Helms (1981: 253) found support for the 'idea that possession of certain racial identity attitudes influences black people's acceptance of black counselors [and other professionals]'. Thus, pre-encounter attitudes 'tended to be associated with pro-white, anti-black counselor preferences' (1981: 254).

The black client may be over-eager to identify with the white worker in order to seek approval. Most individuals at the pre-encounter stage will find attempts to explore racial identity or to focus upon feelings very threatening. Social workers and counselors (black or white) need to help the client to sort out conflicts related to racial/cultural identity. The black social worker can take a nonjudgemental stance toward the client and provide a positive black role model. The white worker, on the other hand, needs to communicate positive attitudes about black people and culture. Both black and white social workers need to guard against unknowingly reinforcing the black client's self-deprecating attitude toward himself/herself and other black people.

Black clients at the encounter stage are more racially aware than pre-encounter clients and are likely to prefer to work with social workers who possess a good knowledge of the client's cultural group. Parham and Helms (1981: 255) found that 'encounter and immersion-emersion attitudes were associated with pro-black, anti-white counselor [and service provide] preferences'. Clients at the encounter stage are preoccupied by questions concerning their concept of self, identity and self-esteem. White social workers and counsellors should capitalize on the black client's motivation toward self-exploration and help the client deal with his or her identity conflicts.

Black clients at the immersion-emersion stage are usually suspicious and hostile towards white professionals. They are likely to regard their psychological problems as products of oppression and racism. In this stage black clients are likely to believe that 'openness or self-disclosure to [white workers] other than one's own [black] group is dangerous because white [professionals] are enemies and members of the oppressing group' (Sue and Sue, 2003, 1990: 110). A white worker will be viewed by the black client as a 'symbol of the oppressive Establishment. If the worker becomes defensive and personalizes the "attacks", he or she will lose his or her effectiveness in [counselling] with the client'. Black clients in the immersion-emersion stage will constantly test the sincerity and openness of the white worker.

A black client in the immersion stage is likely to share his or her problems only with a black worker. However, an immersion client may be anxious that the black worker will not meet his or her standards of blackness. Since the black worker's education, training, authority and status require participation in the white world, the client might believe that these achievements are an indication that the worker is 'psychologically invested' in the world that he or she is rejecting. Parham and Helms (1981: 256) point out that positive therapeutic work can result if the 'client's perception of the therapist are worked through in the initial stages of therapy'. This also applies to the social worker-client relationship.

Some authors have noted unwillingness by blacks with high levels of immersion-emersion attitudes to use mental health services. For instance, Austin *et al.* (1990) suggest that people with high levels of immersion-emersion attitudes may believe that seeing a counselor is stigmatizing and reflects personal weakness. At the internalization stage, black clients may prefer a black social worker but they are also receptive to white social workers as long as the white workers can share, understand and accept their worldviews. Parham and Helms (1981: 255) found that 'internalization attitudes were not strongly related to preferences for a counselor of either race [black or white]'. It appears that as the black client becomes more comfortable with his or her racial identity, the 'race' of the service provider becomes less important. Thus, in order to understand black people's behaviour, white practitioners need 'to search beyond black people's racial self-designation' (Helms, 1981: 255).

The racial identity development model serves as a useful assessment tool for white and black social workers to gain a better understanding of their black clients (Helms, 1986) and themselves, and to communicate in an effective manner. Some scholars have considered the acculturation model (see Chapter 5) to describe and understand the role that culture may play in the therapeutic process. For example, Berry and Kim (1988) suggest that a client's level of acculturation can play an important role in his or her experience of mental health services.

Due to the limitations of a Eurocentric perspective in the diagnosis and treatment of black people's mental disorders, I believe that there is a need for black psychologists and social workers, with the collaboration of other black people, to create and develop their own theories, models, techniques, and institutions for coping with the mental health problems of black people in the UK. The situation in the US is somewhat different from that in Britain 'for there appears to be some recognition of the importance for psychiatry and psychology to be aware of the cultural diversity of its people … "cultural psychiatry" is a well-recognised branch of psychiatry' (Fernando, 2002: 123). Black people in the UK 'have a predominantly negative view about psychiatry and related institutions … [and consider] that the available resources in the mental health field are inappropriate to their needs but that no alternative exists for those in need' (Francis *et al.*, 1993: 143).

Social workers need to be aware that the discrimination that is experienced by people with mental health problems can be intensified if that person happens to be from a black and minority ethnic community (Golightley, 2004). This is illustrated by the following quote from a black person's experience of mental health services: 'coming to mental

health services was like the last straw ... you come to the services dis-
empowered already, they strip you of your dignity ... you become the
dregs of society' (*Keating et al.* 2002: 18).

Various authors argue that black and minority ethnic people continue to struggle to find services that provide them with choice and
control (see Butt and Dhaliwal, 2005 and Chahal, 2004). Graham
observes that the 'colour blind approach has been a constant feature of
the welfare state because of its commitment to provide a universal service where everyone has equal access to the same service' (2007: 112).
Thus 'the services which the welfare state provides have often been
designed from the point of view of dominant groups of people within
society' (Lester and Glasby, 2006: 178). Some authors have called
for improved mental health services for black people because of 'the
perceived "cultural encapsulation" of available mental health services.
Cultural encapsulation involves the chauvinistic and inflexible use of a
worldview or set of cultural values incongruent with the client group
being served .... These perspectives are based on etic (i.e. universal)
assumptions that everyone is similar in their display of behaviours (see
Chapter 1 of this book) related to psychosocial functioning and that
therapeutic change processes are identical and equally effective across
different cultural groups' (Belgrave and Allison, 2005: 292).

Black voluntary organizations have taken the initiative in providing alternative services and treatment for black people. Agencies like
the Afro-Caribbean Mental Health Association and Nafsiyat have
pioneered new practices which recognize the unique social position
of black communities in Britain. As previously mentioned, Nafsiyat
makes psychotherapy available to black clients who are normally
considered linguistically or intellectually incapable of benefiting from
psychotherapy (Kareem and Littlewood, 1999).

8 Conclusion

In this book I have attempted to introduce social workers to the black perspective in psychology, and to describe how this perspective is reflected in education, mental health, identity issues, impression formation, family, and group dynamics. All the chapters stress that social workers' assessment of black clients should focus on understanding the black person's competencies and strengths. The fundamental assumption is that black people are competent, adequate, and different, and not inherently deficient or maladjusted. There is a need for social workers to build on the existing values and strengths in the black community. This approach offers an alternative to the deficit model.

A Eurocentric perspective in psychology has meant certain theoretical deficits when social workers attempt to apply them in practice. As traditional psychology perpetuates a notion of deviance with respect to black people, social workers may be prone to making certain assumptions in their assessments on the basis of these stereotypes. An alternative to focusing on stereotypes or pathological characteristics of black groups is to emphasize the black client's cultural assets and strengths.

This book has presented a perspective that can increase our effectiveness in working with black people. The central theme in this book is the development of a black perspective in psychology and the implications for social work practice. In Britain very little research has been carried out on developing a black perspective in psychology. Much of the existing work on this subject has come from America. This book is intended as an introduction to some of the main principles of a black perspective in psychology. It is my hope that it will inspire discussion and debate in the social work field.

In this book I have argued that social workers need an understanding of the black perspective in psychology in order to be able to deliver effective services to black clients and communities. The social work profession needs to examine and analyse how its methods and approaches, assumptions and assessments, intervention and planning affect black clients. I have argued that traditional psychological principles and theories have not had sufficient explanatory power to account for the behaviour of blacks.

It must be remembered that the major forces that stimulated the growth of a black perspective in psychology were the failure of traditional psychology to provide a full and accurate understanding of black reality, and the pathologization of black people resulting from applications of Eurocentric norms. Psychological practices in Britain and the United States have been white dominated and are often culturally biased and racist. Although white psychologists claimed that they were objective scientists, they define black people from a point of view that focused on defectiveness and pathology. A black perspective in psychology challenges Eurocentric theoretical formulations and research paradigms that have a potentially oppressive effect on black people. It attempts to build a theoretical model that organizes, explains, and leads to understanding the behaviour of black people. In recent years black psychology has become part of a larger movement in psychology – cross-cultural psychology (Belgrave and Allison, 2005; Jones, 2004).

There is a need in Britain for black psychologists and researchers to concentrate on developing paradigms and models that will more accurately depict the reality of black experience.

The traditional method of studying black families in the social science literature has often focused on the pathological rather than on the strengths of black family. Social workers need to mobilize the strengths and competence in black families. Most black researchers agree that the characteristics that help black families to develop, survive, and improve are consistent with Hill's (1972, 1999) analysis of black family strengths. These strengths include strong kinship bonds, strong work orientation, strong achievement orientation, adaptability of family roles, and a strong religious orientation. Hill's work stressed the importance of not viewing differences as pathological, and the importance of helping the many different family structures to function as healthily as possible. This is not to deny that black families face real problems, but it is to build recognition of cultures of strength and resistance to racism into the mainstream of social science and social work theories and models.

Achieving a positive black identity in the face of a racist and oppressive society represents a significant challenge for most black people. Social workers must help black children and youth to master the developmental task of achieving a positive black identity development. The body of research which focuses on models of psychological nigrescence will enable social workers to gain a better understanding of the difficulties experienced by black children, teenagers, and adults in Britain. Other approaches to the study of black identity development include ethnic identity formation theory and acculturation theory.

I have discussed the different perspectives (Eurocentric and black) which have sought to define black people's mental health problems. I have argued that Eurocentric standards of mental health are often inappropriate for black people because they are based on the philosophies, values, and mores of Euro-American culture, and these variables are used to develop normative standards of mental health. We must also question the validity and usefulness of white-originated theories in the treatment of black people. I have argued that we need to develop new definitions of mental health and illness, which reflect a black perspective.

The black perspective on issues critical to the educational achievement of black children is presented in this book. I have discussed the main factors affecting academic success. The educational system must recognize black children's strengths, abilities, and culture, and incorporate them into the learning process.

In this book I have addressed some of the essential components of group work with black people. I have argued that group work theory, practice, and research have traditionally been devoted to the development of universal conceptualizations which can supposedly guide all group practice. This perspective has resulted in most researchers and practitioners ignoring the impact of member and leader ethnicity on group process and outcomes.

Finally, as I have stressed throughout the book, it is imperative that the black perspective in psychology become an integral part of the social work curriculum. It is my hope that the black perspective in psychology will assume a central focus in social work training.

Bibliography

Aalberts, M. L. and Kamminga, E. M. (1983) *Politie en Allochtonen*, Den Haag: Staatsdrukkerij.

Aboud, F. E. and Skerry, S. A. (1984) 'The development of ethnic attitudes: a review', *Journal of Cross-Cultural Psychology*, 15: 3–34.

ABSWAP (1983) *Black Children in Care – Evidence to the House of Commons Social Services Committee*, London: Association of Black Social Workers and Allied Professionals.

Adams, P. L. (1970) 'Dealing with racism in biracial psychiatry', *Journal of the American Academy of Child Psychiatry*, 9, 1: 33–4.

Adebimpe, V. (1981) 'Overview: white norms in psychiatric treatment', *American Journal of Psychiatry*, 138, 3: 275–85.

Adebimpe, V. (1994) 'Race, Racism, and Epidemiological Surveys', *Hospital and Community Psychiatry*, 45, 1: 27–31.

Adelson, J. A. (1953) 'A study of minority group of authoritarianism', *Journal of Abnormal and Social Psychology*, 48: 477–85.

Ahmad, B. (1989) 'Child care and ethnic minorities', in B. Kahan (ed.) *Child Care Research, Policy and Practice*, Milton Keynes: Open University Press.

Ahmad, B. (1990) *Black Perspectives in Social Work*, Birmingham: Venture Press.

Ahmed, S. (1981) 'Asian girls and culture conflict,' in J. Cheetham, W. James, M. Loney, B. Major and W. Prescott (eds.) *Social and Community Work in Multi-Racial Society*, Milton Keynes: Open University Press.

Ahmed, S. (1986) 'Cultural racism in work with Asian women and girls', in S. Ahmed, J. Cheetham, and J. Small (eds.) *Social Work with Black Children and their Families*, London: Batsford.

Ahmed, S. (2005) 'What is the evidence of early intervention, preventative services for black and minority ethnic group?', *Practice*, 7, 2: 89–102.

Aiello, J. and Jones, S. (1971) 'Field study of the proxemic behavior of young school children in three subcultural groups', *Journal of Personality and Social Psychology*, 19: 351–6.

Akbar, N. (1975) 'The rhythm of black personality', *Southern Exposure*, 3: 14–19.

Akbar, N. (1977) *Natural Psychology and Human Transformation*, Chicago, IL: World Community of Islam.

Akbar, N. (1981a) 'Awareness: the key to black mental health', *Journal of Black Psychology*, 1, 1: 30–7.

Akbar, N. (1981b) 'Mental disorder among African Americans', *Black Books Bulletin*, 7, 2: 18–25.

Akbar, N. (1984) *Chains and Images of Psychological Theory*, Chicago, IL: Third World Press.

Akbar, N. (1991) 'Mental disorder among African Americans', in R. L. Jones (ed.) *Black Psychology*, 3rd edn, Berkeley, CA: Cobb & Henry.

Akbar, N. (2004) 'The evolution of human psychology for African Americans', in R. L. Jones (ed.) *Black Psychology*, 4th edn, Berkeley, CA: Cobb & Henry.

Alexander, C. (2000) *The Asian Gang: Ethnicity, Identity, Masculinity*, Oxford and New York: Berg.

Ali, S. and Atkin, K. (2004) *Primary Healthcare and South Asian Populations: Meeting the Challenges*, Oxford: Radcliffe Medical Press.

Andrews, V. L. and Majors, R. G. (2004) 'African American nonverbal culture', in R. L. Jones (ed.) *Black Psychology*, 4th edn, Berkeley, CA: Cobb & Henry.

Anwar, M. (1978) *Between Two Cultures*, London: CRC.

Anwar, M. (1998) *Between Two Cultures*, 2nd edn, London: CRC.

Archer, J. and Lloyd, B. (1982) *Sex and Gender*, Harmondsworth: Penguin.

Argyle, M. (1988) *Bodily Communication*, 2nd edn, London: Methuen.

Asante, M. K. (1980) 'International/intercultural relations', in M. Asante and A. Vandi (eds.) *Contemporary Black Thought*, Beverly Hills, CA: Sage Publications.

Asante, M. K. and Noor-Aldee, H. S. (1984) 'Social interaction of black and white college students', *Journal of Black Studies*, 14: 507–16.

Atkinson, D. R., Morten, G. and Sue, D. W. (1979) *'Counselling American Minorities: A Cross-Cultural Perspective'*, Dubuque, IA: William C. Brown.

Atkinson, D. R., Morten, G. and Sue, D. W. (1979) *'Counselling American Minorities: A Cross-Cultural Perspective'*, Dubuque, IA: McGraw Hill.

Austin, L. N., Carter, R. T. and Vaux, A. (1990) 'The role of racial identity in black students' attitudes toward counseling and counseling centers', *Journal of College Student Development*, 31, 3: 237–43.

Azibo, D. A. (1983) 'Some psychological concomitants and consequences of the Black personality: mental health implications', *Journal of Non-White Concerns in Personnel and Guidance*, 11, 2: 59–66.

Azibo, D. A. (1984) 'Advances in Black personality theory', paper presented at *The 17th Annual Convention of the Association of Black Psychologists*, New York, August.

Azibo, D. A. (1989) 'African-centered theses on mental health and a nosology of Black/African personality disorder', *Journal of Black Psychology*, 15, 2: 173–214.

Bagley, C. (1993) *International and Transracial Adoptions: a Mental Health Perspective*, Aldershot: Avebury.

Bagley, C. and Verma, G. K. (eds.) (1982) *Self-Concept, Achievement and Multi-Cultural Education*, London: Macmillan.

Bagley, C., Bart, M. and Wong, J. (1979) 'Antecedents of scholastic success in West Indian ten-year-olds in London', in G. Verma and C. Bagley (eds.) *Race, Education and Identity*, London: Macmillan.

Bagley, C., Mallick, K. and Verma, G. K. (1979) 'Pupil self-esteem: a study of black and white teenagers in British schools', in G. Verma and C. Bagley (eds.) *Race, Education and Identity*, London: Macmillan.

Bains, J. (2005) 'Race, Culture and Psychiatry', *A History of Transcultural Psychiatry*, 16: 39–154.

Baldwin, J. A. (1976) 'Black psychology and black personality', *Black Books Bulletin* 4, 3: 6–11.

Baldwin, J. A. (1979) 'Theory and research concerning the notion of black self-hatred: a review and reinterpretation', *Journal of Black Psychology*, 5: 51–78.

Baldwin, J. A. (1980) 'The psychology of oppression', in M. K. Asante and A. Vandi (eds.) *Contemporary Black Thought*, Beverly Hills, CA: Sage Publications.

Baldwin, J. A. (1981) 'Notes on an Africentric theory of black personality', *Western Journal of Black Studies*, 5: 172–9.

Baldwin, J. A. (1984) 'African self-consciousness and the mental health of African-Americans', *Journal of Black Studies*, 15, 2: 177–94.

Baldwin, J. A. (1985) 'African self-consciousness: an Afrocentric questionnaire', *Western Journal of Black Studies*, 9, 2: 61–8.

Baldwin, J. A. (1991) 'African (Black) psychology: issues and synthesis', in R. Jones (ed.) *Black Psychology*, 3rd edn, Berkeley, CA: Cobb & Henry.

Baldwin, J. and Hopkins, R. (1990) 'African-American and European-American cultural differences as assessed by the worldviews paradigm: an empirical analysis', *The Western Journal of Black Studies*, 14, 1: 38–52.

Ballard, C. (1979) 'Conflict, continuity and change: second-generation South Asians', in V. Khan (ed.) *Ethnic Minority Families in Britain*, London: Routledge & Kegan Paul.

Banks, G. P., Berenson, B. G. and Carkhoff, R. R. (1967) 'The effects of counselor race and training upon counseling process with Negro clients in initial interviews', *Journal of Clinical Psychology*, 23: 70–2.

Banks, J. A. (1984) 'Black youths in predominantly white suburbs: an exploratory study of their attitudes and self-concepts', *Journal of Negro Education*, 53, 1: 3–17.

Banks, N. (1992) 'Techniques for direct identity work with Black children', *Adoption and Fostering*, 16, 3: 19–25.

Banks, N. (2001) 'Assessing the children and families who belong to minority ethnic groups', in J. Horwath (ed.) *The Child's World*, London; Jessica Kingsley Publishers.

Banks, N. (2002) 'What is black identity?', in Dwivedi, K.N. (ed) *Meeting the Needs of Ethnic Minority Children: A Handbook for Professionals*, 2nd edn, London: Jessica Kingsley Publishers.

Banks, N. (2003) 'What is a positive black identity?', in K. N. Dwivedi (ed.) *Meeting the Needs of Ethnic Minority Children: Including Refugee, Black and Mixed Parentage Children: A Handbook for Professionals*, London: Jessica Kingsley Publishers.

Banks, W. (1972) 'The black client and the helping professional', in R. Jones (ed.) *Black Psychology*, New York: Harper & Row.

Banks, W. (1976) 'White preference in blacks: a paradigm in search of a phenomenon', *Psychological Bulletin*, 83: 1179–86.

Banks, W. C. (1982) 'Deconstructive falsification: foundations of a critical method in Black psychology', in E. Jones and S. Korchin (eds.) *Minority Mental Health*, New York: Praeger.

Banks, W. and Grambs, J. (1972) *Black Self Concept*, New York: McGraw-Hill.

Baratz, S. and Baratz, J. (1970) 'Early childhood intervention: the social science base of institutional racism', *Harvard Educational Review*, 40: 29–50.

Barn, R., Ferdinand, D. and Sinclair, R. (1997) *Acting on Principle: An Examination of Race and Ethnicity in Social Services Provision for Children and Families*, London: British Agencies for Adoption and Fostering.

Barn, R. (2001) *Black Youth on the Margins*, London: Joseph Rowntree Foundation.

Barn, R. (2002) 'Race', ethnicity and child welfare', in B. Mason and A. Sawyer (eds.) *Explaining the Unsaid*, London: Karnac.

Barn, R. (2006) *Parenting in Multiracial Britain*, London: Joseph Rowntree Foundation.

Barnes, E. J. (1972) 'Cultural retardation or shortcomings of assessment techniques?', in R. Jones (ed.) *Black Psychology*, New York: Harper & Row.

Barnes, E. J. (1981) 'The black community as a source of positive self-concept for Black children: a theoretical perspective', in R. L. Jones (ed.) *Black Psychology*, 2nd edn, New York: Harper & Row.

Barnes, E. J. (1991) 'The black community as a source of positive self-concept for Black children: a theoretical perspective', in R. L. Jones (ed.) *Black Psychology*, 3rd edn, Berkeley, CA: Cobb & Henry.

Barnlund, D. (1968) *Interpersonal Communication: Surveys and Studies*, Boston, MA: Houghton Mifflin.

Baron, R. A. and Byrne, D. (1991) *Social Psychology: Understanding Human Interaction*, 6th edn, London: Allyn & Bacon.

Baron, R. A., Byrne, D. and Branscombe, (2005) *Social Psychology: Understanding Human Interaction*, 11th edn, London: Allyn & Bacon.

Baskin, D., Bluestone, H. and Nelson, M. (1981) 'Ethnicity and psychiatric diagnosis', *Journal of Clinical Psychology*, 39: 529–37.

Baugh, J. (1983) *Black Street Speech: Its History, Structure and Survival*, Austin, TX: University of Texas Press.

Baughman, E. E. (1971) *Black Americans*, New York: Academic Press.

Bavington, J. and Majid, A. (1986) 'Psychiatric services for ethnic minority groups', in J. L. Cox (ed.) *Transcultural Psychiatry*, London: Croom Helm.

Beez, W. V. (1969) 'Influence of biased psychological reports on teacher behavior and pupil performance', *Proceedings of the 76th Annual Conventions of the American Psychological Association*, 3: 605–6.

Belgrave, F. and Allison, K. (2005) *African American Psychology*, Thousand Oaks, CA: Sage Publications.

Beliappa, J. (1991) *Illness or Distress? Alternative Models of Mental Health*, London: Confederation of Indian Organisations.

Bernard, S. (2001) *Constructing Lived Experiences: Representations of Black Mothers in Child Sexual Abuse Discourses*, Aldershot: Ashgate Publishing.

Bernstein, B. (1961) 'Social structure, language and learning', *Educational Research*, 3, 3: 163–76.

Berry, J. W. (1969) 'On cross-cultural comparability', *International Journal of Psychology*, 4: 119–28.

Berry, J. W. (1974) 'Psychological aspects of cultural pluralism', *Culture Learning*, 2: 17–22.

Berry, J. W. (1980) Acculturation as adaptation, in A. M. Padilla (ed.) *Acculturation, Theory, Model and Some New Findings*, Boulder, CO: Westview.

Berry, J. W. (1990) 'Psychology of acculturation', in J. Berman (ed.) *Cross-Cultural Perspectives, Nebraska Symposium on Motivation, Vol. 37*, Lincoln, NE: University of Nebraska Press.

Berry, J. W. (1997) 'Immigration, acculturation and adaptation', in J. W. Berry, M. H. Segall and C. Kagitcibasi (eds.) *Handbook of Cross-Cultural Psychology*, 2nd edn, Boston: Allyn & Bacon.

Berry, J. W. and Dasen, P. R. (1974) *Culture and Cognition: Readings in Cross-Cultural Psychology*, London: Methuen.

Berry, J. W. and Kim, U. (1988) 'Acculturation and mental health', in P. R. Dasen, J. W. Berry and N. Sartorius (eds.) *Health and Cross-cultural Psychology: Towards Applications*, Beverly Hills, CA: Sage Publications.

Berry, J. W. and Sam, D. (1997) 'Acculturation and adaptation', in J. W. Berry, M. H. Segall and C. Kagitcibasi (eds.) *Handbook of Cross-cultural Psychology, Vol.3*, 2nd edn, Boston, MA: Allyn & Bacon.

Berry, J. W., Kim, U., Minde, T. and Mok, D. (1987) 'Comparative studies of acculturative stress', *International Migration Review*, 21: 491–511.

Berry, J. W., Kim, U., Power, S., Young, M. and Bujaki, M. (1989) 'Acculturation attitudes in plural societies', *Applied Psychology: An International Review*, 38: 185–206.

Berry, J. W., Poortinga, Y. H., Segall, H. and Dasen, P. R. (1992) *Cross-cultural Psychology: Research and Applications*, Cambridge: Cambridge University Press.

Bhugra, D. and Bhui, K. (1997) 'Cross-cultural psychiatric assessment', *Advances in Psychiatric Treatment*, 3: 103–10.

Bhugra, D. and Bhui, K. S. (1999) 'Racism in psychiatry: paradigm lost, paradigm regained', *International Review of Psychiatry*, 11: 236–43.

Bhugra, D., Corridan, B., Rudge, S. (1999) 'Early manifestations, personality traits and pathways into care for Asian and white first-onset cases of schizophrenia', *Social Psychiatry and Psychiatric Epidemiology*, 34: 595–9.

Bhugra, D. and Cochrane, R. (2001) *Psychiatry in Multicultural Britain*, London: Gaskell.

Bhui, K., Strathdee, K. and Sufraz, R. (1993) 'Asian Inpatients in a District Psychiatric Unit: an Examination of Presenting Features and Routes Into Care', *International Journal of Social Psychiatry*, 39, 3: 208–20.

Bhui, K., Stansfeld S. A., Hull, S., Priebe, S., Mole, F., Feder, G. (2003) 'Ethnic variations in pathways to specialist mental health care: a systematic review', *British Journal of Psychiatry*, 182: 5–16

Bhui, K. (2002) *Racism and Mental Health*, London: Jessica Kingsley Publishers.

Billingsley, A. (1968) *Black Families in White America*, Englewood Cliffs, NJ: Prentice-Hall.

Billingsley, A. (1992) *Climbing Jacob's ladder: The enduring legacy of African American families*, New York: Simon & Schuster.

Billingsley, A. and Giovannoni, J. M. (1970) *'Children of the Storm: Black Children and American Child Welfare*, New York: Harcourt Brace Jovanovich.

Birdwhistell, R. L. (1963) 'The kinesic level in the investigation of emotion', in P. H. Knapp (ed.) *Expression of the Emotions in Man*, New York: International Universities Press.

Blanck, P. D. (1993) 'Interpersonal Expectations in the Courtroom: Studying judges' and juries' behaviour', in P. D. Blanck (ed.). *Interpersonal Expectations Theory, Research and Applications*, Cambridge: Cambridge University Press.

Blauner, R. (1969) 'Internal colonialism and ghetto revolt', *Social Problems*, 16, 4: 393–408.

Bloch, J. B. (1968) 'The white worker and the Negro client in psychotherapy', *Social Work*, 13, 2: 36–42.

Block, C. (1980) 'Black Americans and the cross-cultural counseling experience', in A. J. Marsella and Pederson, P. B. (eds.) *Cross-Cultural Counseling and Psychotherapy*, New York: Pergamon.

Blubaugh, J. A. and Pennington, D. L. (1976) *Crossing Difference: Interracial Communication*, Columbus, OH: Merrill.

Bornstein, M. H. (ed) (1995) *Handbook of Parenting*, Vol. 2, NJ: Lawrence Erlbaum Associates.

Boulton, M. J. and Smith, P. B. (1992) 'The social nature of play fighting and play chasing: Mechanisms and strategies underlying cooperation and compromise', in J. H. Barkow, L. Cosmides and J. Tooby (eds.) *The Adapted Mind*, New York: Oxford University Press.

Bowman, P. J. and Howard, C. (1985) 'Race-related socialization, motivation, and academic achievement: A study of black youths in three-generation families', *Journal of the American Academy of Child Psychiatry*, 24: 134–41.

Boyd-Franklin, N. (1989) *Black Families in Therapy*, London: Guilford Press.

Boyd-Franklin, N. (2003) *Black Families in Therapy*, 2nd edn, London: Guilford Press.

Boyd-Franklin, N. (2004) *From Brotherhood to Manhood: How Black Men Rescue their Relationships and Dreams from the Invisibility Syndrome*, NJ: John Wiley & Sons.

Boyd-Franklin, N., Franklin, A. J. and Toussaint, P. (2001) *Boys into Men: Raising Our African American Teenage Sons*, New York: Plume.

Boykin, A. W. (1981) 'Research directions of Black psychologists', *paper presented at University of Maryland*, April.

Boykin, A. W. (1994) 'Afrocultural expression and its implications for schooling', in E. Hollins, J. King and W. Hayman (eds.) *Teaching Diverse Populations: Formulating a Knowledge Base*, Albany, NY: SUNY Press.

Boykin, A. W. (1997) *Culture Matters in the Psychosocial Experiences of African Americans: Some Conceptual, Process and Practical Considerations*, unpublished manuscript.

Boykin, A. W. and Toms, F. D. (1985) 'Black child socialization; A conceptual framework', in H. P. McAdoo and J. L. McAdoo (eds.) *Black Children: Social, Educational and Parental Environments*, Beverly Hills, CA: Sage Publications.

Brand, E. S., Ruiz, R. A. and Padilla, A. M. (1974) 'Ethnic identification and preference: a review', *Psychological Bulletin*, 81, 2: 860–90.

Brayboy, T. (1971) 'The black patient in group therapy', *International Journal of Group Psychotherapy*, 2, 3: 288–93.

Brayboy, T. (1974) 'Black and white groups and therapists', in D. Milman and G. Goldman (eds.) *Group Process Today: Evaluation and Perspective*, Springfield, IL: Charles C. Thomas.

Brigham, J. C. (1974) 'Views of black and white children concerning the distribution of personality characteristics', *Journal of Personality*, 42: 144–58.

Brislin, R. and Yoshida, T. (1994) *Intercultural Communication Training: An Introduction*, Thousand Oaks, CA: Sage Publications.

Broad, B. (2001) *Kinship Care: The Placement Choice for Children and Young People*, Dorset: Russell House Publishing.

Brown, C. (1984) *Black and White in Britain: The Third PSI Survey*, London: Heinemann.

Bryan, B., Dadzie, S. and Scafe, S. (1985) *The Heart of the Race: Black Women's Lives in Britain*, London: Virago.

Burkard, A. W., Juarez-Huffaker, M. and Ajmere, K. (2003) 'White racial identity attitudes as a predictor of client perceptions of cross-cultural working alliances', *Journal of Multicultural Counseling and Development*, 31: 226–36.

Burlew, K. (1979) 'An expectancy approach to understanding black motivation and achievement', in W. D. Smith, K. Burlew, M. Mosley and W. Whitney (eds.) *Reflections on Black Psychology*, Washington, DC: University Press of America.

Butt, J. and Dhaliwal, S. (2005) *Different Paths: Challenging Services*. London: Habinteg Housing Association.

Byers, P. and Byers, H. (1972) 'Nonverbal communication and the education of children', in C. B. Cazden, V. P. John and D. Hymes (eds.) *Functions of Language in the Classroom*, New York: Academic Press.

Campbell, B. and Rose, J. (1992) 'Language and race', *The Journal of Training and Development*, 2, 4: 14–20.

Campling, P. (1989) 'Race, culture and psychotherapy', *Psychiatric Bulletin*, 13: 550–1.

Carpenter, L. and Brockington, I. F. (1980) 'A study of mental illness in Asians, West Indians and Africans living in Manchester', *British Journal of Psychiatry*, 137: 201–5.

Carter, J. H. (1974) 'Recognizing psychiatric symptoms in black Americans', *Geriatrics*, 29: 95–9.

Carter, R. T. (1995) *The Influence of Race and Racial Identity in Psychotherapy*, New York: John Wiley & Sons.

Carter, R. and Helms, J. (1990) 'White racial identity attitudes and cultural values', in J. Helms (ed.) *Black and White Racial Identity: Theory, Research and Practice*, New York: Greenwood Press.

Cashmore, E. (1979) *Rastaman*, London: Allen & Unwin.

Cassen, R. and Kingdon, G. (2007) *Tackling Low Educational Achievement*, London: Joseph Rowntree Foundation.

Cazenave, N. A. (1979) 'Middle-income black fathers: an analysis of the provider role', *Family Coordinator*, 28: 583–93.

CCETSW (1991a) *Dip SW: Rules and Requirements for the Diploma in Social Work*, London: CCETSW.

CCETSW (1991b) *One Small Step Towards Racial Justice: The Teaching of Antiracism in Diploma in Social Work*, London: CCETSW.

CCETSW (1991c) *The Teaching of Child Care in the Diploma in Social Work*, London: CCETSW.

Census (2001) http://www.statistics.gov.uk/.

Centre for Educational Research (2003) http://www.dfes.gov.uk/exclusions/.

Chahal, K. (2004) *Experiencing Ethnicity: Discrimination and Service Provision*, York: Joseph Rowntree Foundation.

Chaplin, P. (1975) *Dictionary of Psychology*, New York: Dell.

Cheek, D. (1976) *Assertive Black Puzzled White: A Black Perspective on Assertive Behaviour*, Berkeley, CA: Impact Publishers.

Chen, M. and Han, Y.S. (2001). 'Cross-cultural group counseling with Asians: A stage-specific interactive approach', *Journal of Specialist in Group Work*, 26: 111–28.

Chivers, T. S. (1987) *Race and Culture in Education*, Windsor: NFER-Nelson.

Chu, J. and Sue, S. (1984) 'Asian/Pacific-Americans and group practice', *Social Work with Groups*, 7: 23–36.

Claiborn, W. L. (1969) 'Expectancy effects in the classroom: a failure to replicate', *Journal of Educational Psychology*, 60: 377–83.

Clark, C. (1971) 'General systems theory and Black studies: some points of convergence', in C. Thomas (ed.) *Boys, No More*, Encino, CA: Glencoe.

Clark (X), C. (1972) 'Black studies or the study of black people', in R. Jones (ed.) *Black Psychology*, New York: Harper & Row.

Clark, K. (1965) *Dark Ghetto*, New York: Harper & Row.

Clark, K. and Clark, M. (1939) 'The development of consciousness of self and the emergence of racial identification in Negro pre-school children', *Journal of Social Psychology*, 10: 591–9.

Clark, K. and Clark, M. (1940) 'Skin color as a factor in racial identification of Negro preschool children', *Journal of Social Psychology*, 11: 159–69.

Clark, K. and Clark, M. (1947) 'Racial identification and preference in Negro children', in T. M. Newcomb and E. L. Hartley (eds.) *Readings in Social Psychology*, New York: Holt.

Clark, K. and Clark, M. (1950) 'Emotional factors in racial identification and preference in Negro children', *Journal of Negro Education*,19: 341–50.

Clark, K. B. (1965) *Dark Ghetto*, New York: Harper & Row.

Clark, L., Swim, J. K. and Cross, W.E. (1995) *Functions of racial identity in everyday life: A daily diary study*, Unpublished manuscript.

Clark, M. L. (1982) 'Racial group concept and self-esteem in Black children', *Journal of Black Psychology*, 8: 75–88.

Clark, R. (1983) *Family Life and School Achievement,* Chicago, IL: University of Chicago Press.

Clarke, P., Harrison, M., Patel, K., Shah, M., Varley, M. and Zack-Williams, T. (1993) *Improving Mental Health Practice*, Leeds: CCETSW.

Coard, B. (1971) *How the West Indian Child is Made ESN in the British School System,* London: New Beacon Books.

Cochrane, R. (1977) 'Mental illness in immigrants to England and Wales: an analysis of mental hospital admissions', *Social Psychiatry,* 12, 25–35.

Cole, M., Gay, J. A., and Sharp, D. W. (1971) *The Cultural Context of Learning and Thinking: An Exploration in Experimental Anthropology,* New York: Basic Books.

Coleman, J. (1972) *Abnormal Psychology and Modern Life,* 4th edn, Glenview, IL: Scott, Foresman.

Coleman, J. C. and Hendry, L. B. (1999) *The Nature of Adolescence*, London: Routledge.

Comer, J. P. (1972) *Beyond Black and White,* New York: Quadrangle Books.

Comer, J. P. (1980) 'White racism: its root form, and function', in R. L. Jones (ed.) *Black Psychology,* 2nd edn, New York: Harper & Row.

Comer, J. P. and Poussaint, A. F. (1992) *Raising Black Children,* New York: Plume Books.

Commission for Healthcare (2007) 'State of healthcare 2007: improvements and challenges in services in England and Wales', Healthcare Commission, London: Stationery Office.

Cooke, B. (1980) 'Nonverbal communication among Afro-Americans: an initial classification', in R. L. Jones (ed.) *Black Psychology,* 2nd edn, New York: Harper & Row.

Cooley, C. (1956) *Human Nature and the Social Order,* New York: Free Press.

Coombs, R. H. and Davies, V. (1966) 'Self-conception and the relationship between high school and college scholastic achievement', *Sociology and Social Research*, 50: 468–9.

Cox, J. L. (1977) 'Aspects of transcultural psychiatry', *British Journal of Psychiatry*, 130: 211–21.

Cox, J. L. (ed.) (1986) *Transcultural Psychiatry*, London: Croom Helm.

Craft, M. and Craft, A. Z. (1983) 'The participation of ethnic minority pupils in further and higher education', *Educational Research*, 25: 10–17.

Cramer, P. and Anderson, G. (2003). 'Ethnic/racial attitudes and self-identification of black Jamaican and white New England children', *Journal of Cross-cultural Psychology*, 34: 395–416.

Cross, A. (1976) 'The black experience: its importance in the treatment of black clients', *Child Welfare*, 53, 3: 158–86.

Cross, W. E. (1971) 'The Negro to black conversion experience: towards the psychology of black liberation', *Black World*, 20: 13–27.

Cross, W. E. (1978) 'The Thomas and Cross models of psychological nigrescence: a literature review', *The Journal of Black Psychology*, 5, 1: 13–31.

Cross, W. E. (1980) 'Models of psychological nigrescence: a literature review', in R. L. Jones (ed.) *Black Psychology*, 2nd edn, New York: Harper & Row.

Cross, W. E. (1985) 'Black identity: rediscovering the distinction between personal identity and reference group orientation', in M. B. Spencer, G. K. Brookins and W. R. Allen (eds.) *Beginnings: The Social and Affective Development of Black Children*, Hillsdale, NJ: Erlbaum.

Cross, W. E. (1991) *Shades of Black: Diversity in African American Identity*, Philadelphia, PA: Temple University Press.

Cross, W. E. (1995) 'The psychology of nigrescence: revising the Cross model', in J. G. Ponterotto, J. M. Casas, L. A. Suzuki and C. M. Alexander (eds.) *Handbook of Multicultural Counseling*, Thousand Oaks, CA: Sage Publications.

Cross, W. E. (2001). 'Encountering Nigrescence', in J. G. Ponterotto, J.M. Casas, L.A. Suzuki and C.M. Alexander (eds.), *Handbook of Multicultural Counseling*, Thousand Oaks, CA: Sage Publications.

Cross, W. E., Parham, T. A. and Helms, J. E. (1991) 'The stages of black identity development: nigrescence models', in R. L. Jones (ed.) *Black Psychology*, 3rd edn, Berkeley, CA: Cobb & Henry.

Cross, W. E., Parham, T. A. and Helms, J. E. (1995) 'The stages of black identity development: nigrescence models', in R.L. Jones (ed) *Black Psychology*, 2nd edn, Berkeley, CA: Cobb & Henry.

Cross, W.E. and Fhagen-Smith, O. (1996) 'Nigrescence and ego identity development, in P. Petersen, J. Draguns, W. Lonner and J. Trimnle (eds.) *Counseling Across Cultures*, Thousand Oaks, CA: Sage Publications.

Cross, W. E., Parham, T. A. and Helms, J. E. (1998) 'Nigresence revisited: theory and research', in R. L. Jones (ed.) *African American Identity Development*, Hampton, VA: Cobb & Henry.

Cross, W. E., Jr., and Vandiver, B. J. (2001). 'Nigrescence theory and measurement: Introducing the Cross Racial Identity Scale (CRIS)', in J. G. Ponterotto, J. M. Casas, L. A. Suzuki and C. M. Alexander (eds.) *Handbook of Multicultural Counseling* (2nd edn), Thousand Oaks, CA: Sage Publications.

Curran, H. V. (1984) 'Introduction', in H. V. Curran (ed.) *Nigerian Children: Developmental Perspectives,* London: Routledge & Kegan Paul.

Dalal, F. (1988) 'The racism of Jung', *Race and Class*, 29, 3: 1–22.

Dana, D. (1981) *Human Services for Cultural Minorities,* Maryland: Baltimore University Park Press.

D'Andrea, M. and Daniels, J. (2001) 'Expanding our thinking about White racism: Facing the challenge of multicultural counseling in the 21st century', in J. G. Ponterotto, J. M. Casas, L. A. Suzuki, L. A. and C. M. Alexander (eds.), *The Handbook of Multicultural Counseling*, 2nd edn. Thousand Oaks, CA: Sage Publications.

Davey, A. G. (1987) 'Insiders, outsiders and anomalies: a review of studies of identities – a reply to Olivia Foster-Carter', *New Community*, 13, 3: 477–82.

Davey, A. G. and Mullin, P. N. (1980) 'Ethnic identification and preference of British primary school children', *Journal of Child Psychology and Psychiatry*, 21: 241–51.

Davey, A. G. and Norburn, M. V. (1980) 'Ethnic awareness and ethnic differentiations amongst primary school children', *New Community*, 8, 1/2: 51–60.

Davis, L. (1979) 'Racial composition of groups', *Social Work,* 24: 208–13.

Davis, L. (1980) 'Racial balance: a psychological issue', *Social Work with Groups*, 3, 2: 75–85.

Davis, L. (1981) 'Racial issues in training of group workers', *Journal for Specialists in Group Work,* August: 155–60.

Davis, L. (1984) 'Essential components of group work with Black Americans', *Social Work with Groups*, 7: 97–109.

Davis, S. E. (1982) *'Black Psychology',* unpublished manuscript, University of Maryland.

Davison, G. C. and Neale, J. M. (1986) *Abnormal Psychology,* 4th edn, New York: Wiley.

Davison, G. C. and Neale, J. M. (2001) *Abnormal Psychology*, 8th edn, New York; Wiley.

Dean, G., Walsh, H., Downing, H. and Shelly, E. (1981) 'First admissions of native born and immigrants to psychiatric hospitals in south east England 1976', *British Journal of Psychiatry,* 139: 506–12.

Demo, D. H. and Hughes, M. (1990) 'Socialization and racial identity among black Americans', *Social Psychology Quarterly*, 53, 4: 364–74.

Department of Health (2001) *The Children Act Now: Messages from Research*, London: HMSO.

Department of Health (2002) *Requirements for Social Work Training*, London: HMSO.

DES (Department of Education and Science) (1985) see Swann (1985).

Deutsch, M. (1968) 'The disadvantaged child and the learning process', in A. Passou (ed.) *Education in Depressed Areas,* New York: Columbia University Teachers College.

Devore, W. and Schlesinger, E. (1981) *Ethnic-Sensitive Social Work Practice,* St Louis, MO: C. V. Mosby.

Devore, W. and Schlesinger, E. (1998) *Ethnic-Sensitive Social Work Practice,* 5th edn, Boston, MA: Allyn & Bacon.

Dixon, V. and Foster, B. (1971) *Beyond Black or White,* Boston, MA: Little, Brown.

Dodd, I. (1977) *Perspectives on Cross-Cultural Communication,* Dubuque, IA: Kendall/Hunt.

Dodson, J. (1988) 'Conceptualizations of black families', in H. P. McAdoo (ed.) *Black Families,* London: Sage Publications.

Dominelli, L. (1988) *Anti-Racist Social Work,* London: Macmillan.

Dominelli, L. (1992) 'An uncaring profession? An examination of racism in social work', in P. Braham, A. Rattansi, and R. Skellington (eds.) *Racism and Antiracism,* London: Sage Publications.

Dominelli, L. (1997) *Anti-Racist Social Work,* 2nd edn, London: Macmillan.

Donovan, S. and Cross, C. T. (2002) *Minority Students in Special Education and Gifted Education,* Washington: National Academy Press.

Dosanjh, J. S. and Ghuman, P. A. S. (1996) *Child-rearing in Ethnic Minorities,* Clevedon: Multilingual Matters.

Dove, L. (1974) 'Racial awareness among adolescents in London comprehensive schools', *New Community,* 3: 255–61.

Dovidio, J. F., Gaertner, S. L., Kawakami, K. and Hodson, G. (2002). 'Why can't we just get along? Interpersonal biases and interracial distrust', *Cultural Diversity & Ethnic Minority Psychology,* 8: 88–102.

Drew, D. and Gray, J. (1991) 'The black-white gap in examination results: a statistical critique of a decade's research', *New Community,* 17, 2: 159–72.

Driver, G. (1980) *Beyond Underachievement,* London: Commission for Racial Equality.

Driver, G. (1982) 'Ethnicity and cultural competence: aspects of interaction in multi-racial classrooms', in G. K. Verma and C. Bagley (eds.) *Self Concept, Achievement and Multicultural Education,* London: Macmillan.

DuBois, W. E. B. (1908) *The Negro American Family,* Atlanta, GA: Atlanta University Press.

Dukes, R. L. and Martinez, R. (1994) 'The impact of eth-gender on self-esteem among adolescents', *Adolescence,* 29: 105–15.

Duncan, B. L. (1978) 'Nonverbal communication', *Psychological Bulletin,* 72: 118–37.

Dwivedi, K. N. (2002) *Meeting the Needs of Ethnic Minority Children: A Handbook for Professionals,* 2nd edn, London: Jessica Kingsley Publishers.

Eakins, B. and Eakins, G. (1978) *Sex Differences in Human Communication,* Boston, MA: Houghton Mifflin.

Edwards, A. and Polite, C. (1992) *Children of the Dream: The Psychology of Black Success,* New York: Doubleday.

Ekman, P. (1972) 'Universal and cultural differences in facial expression of emotion', in J. K. Cole (ed.) *Nebraska Symposium on Motivation,* Lincoln, NE: University of Nebraska Press.

Ekman, P. and Friesen, W. V. (1967) 'Origin, usage and coding: the basis for five categories of nonverbal behaviour', paper presented at the *Symposium on Communication Theory and Linguistic Models*, Buenos Aires.

Ely, P. and Denny, D. (1989) *Social Work in a Multi-Racial Society*, Aldershot: Ashgate.

Erickson, F. (1976) 'Talking down and giving reasons: hyper-explanation and listening behaviour in inter-racial interviews', paper presented at the *International Conference on Non-verbal Behaviour*, Ontario Institute for Studies in Education, Toronto, Canada.

Erikson, E. H. (1964) 'Memorandum on identity and Negro youth', *Journal of Social Issues*, 20, 4: 29–42.

Erikson, E. H. (1968) *Identity: Youth and Crisis*, London: Faber.

Essed, P. (1990) *Everyday Racism: Reports from Women of Two Cultures*, Claremont, CA: Hunter House.

Fairchild, H. (1988) 'Glorification of things White', *The Journal of Black Psychology*, 14, 2: 73–4.

Fairchild, H. (1991) 'Scientific racism: The cloak of objectivity', *Journal of Social Issues*, 47, 3: 101–15.

Fairchild, H. and Edwards-Evans, S. (1990) 'African American dialects and schooling: a review', in A. M. Padilla, H. H. Fairchild and C. M. Valadez (eds.) *Bilingual Education: Issues and Strategies*, Newbury Park, CA: Sage Publications.

Farmer, E. and Moyers, S. (2005) *Children placed with relatives or friends: placement patterns and outcomes*, Report to the Department for Education and Skills, Bristol: University of Bristol.

Farrell, W. C. and Olson, J. L. (1983) 'Kenneth and Mamie Clark revisited: radical identification and racial preference in dark-skinned and light-skinned black children', *Urban Education*, 18, 3: 284–97.

Fatimilehin, I. (1999) 'Of jewel heritage: Racial socialization and racial identity attitudes among adolescents of mixed African Caribbean/White parentage', *Journal of Adolescence*, 22: 303–18.

Fatimilihein, I. (2002) The Development of Racial and Ethnic Identity in Adolescence, Unpublished PhD Thesis.

Favazza, A. R. and Oman, M. (1978) 'Overview: foundations of cultural psychiatry', *American Journal of Psychiatry*, 135: 293–303.

Fellows, B. (1968) *The Discrimination Process and Development*, Oxford: Pergamon.

Fernando, S. (1988) *Race and Culture in Psychiatry*, London: Croom Helm.

Fernando, S. (2002) *Mental Health, Race and Culture*, Basingstoke: Macmillan.

Fernando, S. (2003) *Cultural Diversity, Mental Health and Psychiatry: The Struggle Against Racism*, London: Routledge.

Fine, M. and Bowers, C. (1984) 'Racial self-identification: the effects of social history and gender', *Journal of Applied Social Psychology*, 14: 136–46.

Fitzherbert, K. (1967) *West Indian Children in London*, London: Bell.

Fleming, E. S. and Anttonen, R. G. (1971) 'Teacher expectancy or my fair lady', *Aera Journal*, 8: 241.

Fong, R. D. (2004) *Culturally Competent Practice with Immigrant and Refugee Children and Families*, New York: Guildford Press.

Foster, H. J. (1983) 'African patterns in the Afro-American family', *Journal of Black Studies*, 14, 2: 201–32.

Foster, P. (1990) *Policy and Practice in Multicultural and Anti-Racist Education*, London: Routledge.

Foster, P. (1992) 'Teacher attitudes and Afro/Caribbean educational attainment', *Oxford Review of Education*, 18, 3: 269–81.

Fowler, B., Littlewood, B. and Madigan, R. (1977) 'Immigrant school leavers and the search for work', *Sociology*, 11, 1: 65–85.

Francis, E. (1991) 'Mental health, antiracism and social work training', in CCETSW *One Small Step Towards Racial Justice*, London: CCETSW.

Francis, E., David, J., Johnson, N. and Sashidaran, S. P. (1993) 'Black people and psychiatry in the UK', in P. Clarke, M. Harrison, K. Patel, M. Shah, M. Varley and T. Zack-Williams (eds.) *Improving Mental Health Practice*, Leeds: CCETSW.

Frazier, E. F. (1939) *The Negro Family in United States*, Chicago, IL: University of Chicago Press.

Freeman, E. M. (1990) 'The Black family's life cycle: operationalizing a strengths perspective', in S. M. Logan, E. M. Freeman and R. G. McRoy (eds) *Social Work Practice with Black Families*, New York: Longman.

Freud, S. (1912–13) *Totem and Taboo*, Harmondsworth: Penguin Freud Library 13.

Fugita, S., Wexley K. and Hillery, J. M. (1974) 'Black-white differences in nonverbal behaviour in an interview setting', *Journal of Applied Social Psychology*, 4: 343–50.

Fuller, M. (1980) 'Black girls in a London comprehensive school', in R. Deem (ed.) *Schooling for Women's Work*, London: Routledge & Kegan Paul.

Gadsden, V. (1999) 'Black families in intergenerational and cultural perspective', in M. E. Lamb (ed.) *Parenting and Child Development in "Nontraditional" Families*, NJ: Lawrence Erlbaum.

Galton, F. (1869) *Hereditary Genius: Its Laws and Consequences*, London: Macmillan.

Gambe, D., Gomes, J., Kapur, V., Rangel, M. and Stubbs, P. (1992) *Improving Practice with Children and Families*, Leeds: CCETSW.

Garcia Coll, C. T., Meyer, E. C. and Brillon, L. (1995) 'Ethnic and minority parenting', in M. H. Bornstein (ed.) *Handbook of Parenting*, Vol 2, Mahwah, NJ: Lawrence Erlbaum Associates.

Garcia Coll, C. T. and Magnuson, K. (1997) 'The psychological experience of immigration: A developmental perspective', in A. Booth, A. C. Crouter and N. Landale (eds.) *Immigration and the Family: Research and Policy on US Immigrants*, Mahwah, NJ: Erlbaum.

Gardner, H. (1993) *Frames of Mind: The Theory of Multiple Intelligences* (10), New York: Basic Books.

Gardiner, H. W. (2004) 'Follow the yellow brick road: New approaches to the study of cross-cultural human development', in V. P. Gielen and J. L.

Roopnarine (eds.) *Childhood and Adolescence: Cross-cultural Applications*, Westport, CT: Greenwood Press.

Gardner, L. H. (1971) 'The therapeutic relationship under varying conditions of race', *Psychotherapy: Theory, Research and Practice* 8, 1: 78–87.

Garratt, G. A., Baxter, J. C., and Rozelle, R. M. (1981) 'Training university police in Black-American nonverbal behaviors', *Journal of Social Psychology*, 113: 217–29.

Garvin, C. (1981) *Contemporary Group Work*, Englewood Cliffs, NJ: Prentice-Hall.

Gatz, M., Tyler, F. and Pargament, A. (1978) 'Goal attainment, locus of control, and coping style in adolescents group counseling', *Journal of Counseling Psychology*, 25, 4: 310–19.

German, G. (2002) 'Antiracist strategies for educational performance: Facilitating successful learning for all children', in K. N. Dwivedi (ed.) *Meeting the Needs of Ethnic Minority Children: Including Refugee, Black and Mixed Parentage Children: A Handbook for Professionals*, London: Jessica Kingsley Publishers.

Ghuman, P. A. S. (1997) 'Assimilation or integration? A study of Asian adolecents', *Educational Research*, 39: 23–35.

Ghuman, P. A. S. (1999) *Asian Adolescents in the West*, Leicester: British Psychological Society.

Ghuman, P. A. S. (2003) *Double Loyalties: South Asian Adolescents in the West*, Cardiff: University of Wales Press.

Gibbs, J. T. (1974) 'Patterns of adaptation among Black students at a predominantly White university: selected case studies', *American Journal of Orthopsychiatry*, 44, 5: 728–40.

Gibson, A. (1986) *The Unequal Struggle*, London: Centre for Caribbean Studies.

Giggs, J. (1986) 'Ethnic status and mental illness in urban areas', in T. Rathwell and D. Phillips (eds.) *Health, Race and Ethnicity*, London: Croom Helm.

Giles, H. and Johnson, P. (1981) 'The role of language in ethnic group relations', in J. Turner and H. Giles (eds.) *Intergroup Behaviour*, Chicago, IL: University of Chicago Press.

Giles, H. and Coupland, N. (1991) *Language: Contexts and Consequences*, Pacific Grove, CA: Brooks/Cole.

Gillborn, D. (1990) *'Race', Ethnicity and Education: Teaching and Learning in Multi-Ethnic Schools*, London: Routledge.

Gillborn, D. (2001) 'Racism, policy and the (mis) education of black children', in Majors, R. (ed.) *Educating Our Black Children*, London: Routledge.

Gillborn, D. and Drew, D. (1992) 'Race, class and school effects', *New Community*, 18, 4: 551–65.

Gillborn, D. and Gipps, C. (1996) *Recent Research on the Achievements of Ethnic Minority Pupils*, London: HMSO.

Gillborn, D. and Mirza, H. (2000) *Educational Inequality: Mapping Race, Class and Gender*, London: OfSTED.

Gillborn, D. and Youdell, D. (2000) *Rationing Education: policy, practice, reform and equity*, Buckinghamshire: Open University Press.

Goffman, E. (1959) *The Presentation of Self in Everyday Life*, Garden City, NY: Doubleday.

Golightley, M. (2004) *Social Work and Mental Health*, Exeter: Learning Matters.

Goodman, M. E. (1946) 'Evidence concerning the genesis of inter-racial attitudes', *American Anthropology*, 48: 624–30.

Goodman, M. E. (1952) *Racial Awareness in Young Children*, Cambridge, MA: Addison Wesley.

Gopaul-McNicol, S. (1988) 'Racial identification and racial preference of black preschool children in New York and Trinidad', *The Journal of Black Psychology*, 14, 2: 65–8.

Gopaul-McNicol, S. (1993) *Working with West Indian Families*, New York: Guilford Press.

Gordon, T. (1973) 'Notes on White and Black psychology', *Journal of Social Issues*, 29, 1: 87–95.

Graham, M. (2000) 'Black issues in social work and social care', *Social Work Education*, 19, 5: 423–36.

Graham, M. (2001) 'The 'miseducation' of Black children in the British educational system – towards an African-centred orientation to knowledge', in R. Majors (ed.) *Educating Our Black Children: New Directions and Radical Approaches*, London: Routledge.

Graham, M. (2007) *Black Issues in Social Work and Social Care*, Bristol: Policy Press.

Graves, T. (1967) 'Psychological acculturation in a tri-ethnic community', *Southwestern Journal of Anthropology*, 23: 337–50.

Green, J. (1982) *Cultural Awareness in the Human Services*, Englewood Cliffs, NJ: Prentice-Hall.

Green, P. A. (1982) 'Teachers' influence on the self-concept of pupils of different ethnic groups', unpublished PhD thesis, University of Durham.

Gregor, A. J. and McPherson, D. A. (1966) 'Racial preferences and ego-identity among white and Bantu children in the Republic of South Africa', *Genetic Psychology Monographs*, 73: 217–53.

Grier, W. and Cobbs, P. (1968) *Black Rage*, New York: Bantam.

Griffith, M. S. (1977) 'The influence of race on the psychotherapeutic relationship', *Psychiatry*, 40, 1: 27–40.

Gudkonsson, G.H., Rabe-Hesketh, S. and Szumkler, G. (2004) 'Management of psychiatric inpatient violence: patient ethnivity and use of medication, restraint and seclusion', *British Journal of Psychiatry*, 184: 258–62.

Gudykunst, W. B. (2004) *Bridging Differences: Effective Intergroup Communication*, London: Sage Publications.

Gudykunst, W. B. and Kim, Y. Y. (1997). *Communicating With Strangers*, New York: McGraw-Hill.

Gullattee, A. C. (1969) 'The Negro psyche: fact, fiction and fantasy', *Journal National Medical Association*, 61: 119–29.

Guthrie, R. V. (1976) *Even the Rat was White: A Historical View of Psychology*, New York: Harper & Row.

Guthrie, R. V. (2003) *Even the Rat was White: A Historical View of Psychology*, New York: Harper & Row.

Guthrie, R. V. (2004) 'The psychology of African Americans: An historical perspective', in R. L. Jones (ed.) *Black Psychology*, 4th edn, Berkeley, CA: Cobb & Henry.

Gynther, M. (1972) 'White norms and black MMPI's: a prescription for discrimination', *Psychological Bulletin*, 78: 386–402.

Gynther, M. and Green, S. B. (1980) 'Accuracy may make a difference, but does a difference make for accuracy? A response to Pritchard and Rosenblatt', *Journal of Consulting and Clinical Psychology*, 48: 268–72.

Halberstadt, A. G. (1985) 'Race, socioeconomic status, and nonverbal behaviour', in A. W. Siegman and S. Feldstein (eds.) *Multichannel Integrations of Nonverbal Behaviour*, Hillsdale, NJ: Lawrence Erlbaum.

Hale, J. E. (1982) *Black Children: Their Routes, Culture and Learning Styles*, Provo, UT: Brigham Young University Press.

Hall, E. T. (1955) 'The anthropology of manners', *Scientific American*, 192: 85–9.

Hall, E. T. (1964) 'Adumbration as a feature of intercultural communication', *American Anthropologist*, 66: 154–63.

Hall, E. T. (1974) *Handbook for Proxemic Research*, Washington, DC: Society for the Anthropology of Visual Communication.

Hall, E. T. (1976) *Beyond Culture*, New York: Anchor Press.

Hall, E. T. (1984) 'The hidden dimensions of time and space in today's world', in F. Poyatos (ed.) *Cross-cultural Perspectives in Nonverbal Communication*, Toronto: C.J. Hogrefe.

Hall, E. T. (1994) 'Monochronic and polychronic time', in L. A. Samovar and R. E. Porter (eds.) *Intercultural Communication: A Reader*, Belmont, CA: Wadsworth.

Hall, S. (1992) 'New ethnicities in "race", culture and difference', in J. Donald and A. Rattansi (eds.) *Open University Reader*, London: Sage Publications.

Hall, W. S., Cross, W. E., Jr. and Freedle, R. (1972) 'Stages in the development of a black identity', *ACT research report 50*, Iowa City, IA: Research and Development Division, American Testing Program.

Halpern, F. (1973) *Survival: Black/White*, New York: Pergamon.

Hanna, J. L. (1984) 'Black/white nonverbal differences, dance and dissonance: implications for desegregation', in A. Wolfgang (ed.) *Nonverbal Behaviour: Perspectives, Applications, Intercultural Insights*, Lewiston, NY: C. J. Hogrefe.

Hanson, B. and Klerman, G. L. (1974) 'Interracial problems in the assessment of clinical depression: concordance differences between white psychiatrists and black and white patients', *Psychopharmacological Bulletin*, 10: 65–6.

Hare, N. and Hare, J. (1984) *The Endangered Black Family*, San Francisco, CA: Black Think Tank.

Harper, R. G., Wiens, A. N. and Matarazzo, J. D. (1978) *Nonverbal Communication*, New York: Wiley.

Harrison, A. O. (1981) 'The Black family's socializing environment', in H. P. McAdoo (ed.) *Black Families*, Beverly Hills, CA: Sage Publications.

Harrison, D. K. (1977) 'The attitudes of Black counselees toward White counselors', *Journal of Non-White Concerns in Personnel and Guidance*, 5, 2: 52–9.

Harrison-Ross, P. and Wyden, B. (1973) *The Black Child – A Parents' Guide*, New York: Peter H. Wyden.

Harvey, A. R. (2005) 'Group work with African American youth in the criminal justice system; A culturally competent model' in G. R. Grief and P. H. Ephross (2005) *Group Work with Populations at Risk*, Oxford: Oxford University Press.

Hayes, W. A. (1980) 'Radical black behaviourism', in R. L. Jones (ed.) *Black Psychology*, 2nd edn, New York: Harper & Row.

Hayles. R. V., Bell, S. R., Evans, W., Floyd, L. J., Monteiro, N., Daniels, I.N. and Harrell, C. J. (2004) 'African American strengths' in R. L. Jones (ed.) *Black Psychology*, 4th edn, New York: Harper & Row.

Haynes, N. (1995) 'How skewed is the Bell curve?', *Journal of Black Psychology*, 21: 275–92.

Hays, W. and Mendel, C. H. (1973) 'Extended kinship relations in black and white families', *Journal of Marriage and the Family*, 35: 51–7.

Heffernon, A. and Bruehl, D. (1971) 'Some effects of race of inexperienced lay counselors on Black junior high school students', *Journal of School Psychology*, 9, 1: 35–7.

Heinig, R. M. (1975) 'A descriptive study of teacher-pupil tactile communication in grades four through six', doctoral dissertation, University of Pittsburgh.

Helms, J. E. (1984) 'Towards a theoretical explanation of the effects of race on counseling: a Black and White model', *The Counseling Psychologist*, 12, 4: 153–65.

Helms, J. E. (1985). 'Cultural identity in the treatment process', in P. Pedersen (ed.), *Handbook of Cross-cultural Counseling and Therapy*, Westport, CT: Greenwood Press.

Helms, J. E. (1986) 'Expanding racial identity theory to cover counseling process', *Journal of Counseling Psychology*, 33, 1: 62–4.

Helms, J. E. (1989) 'Considering some methodological issues in racial identity counseling research', *The Counseling Psychologist*, 17: 227–52.

Helms, J. E. (1990) 'Generalizing racial identity interaction theory to groups', in J. E. Helms (ed.) *Black and White Racial Identity: Theory, Research and Practice*, New York: Greenwood Press.

Helms, J. E. (1993) 'I also said White racial identity influences White researchers', *The Counseling Psychologist*, 21: 240–3.

Helms, J. E. (1995) 'An update of Helms's white and people of color racial identity models', in A. J. Ponterotto, J. M. Casas, L. S. Suzuki and C. M. Alexander (eds.) *Handbook of Multicultural Counseling*, London: Sage Publications.

Helms, J. E. (2003) 'Racial identity and racial socialization as aspects of adolescents' identity development', in R. Lerner, F. Jacobs, and D. Wertlief (eds.) *Handbook of Applied Developmental Science: Promoting Positive Child, Adolescent, and Family Development Through Research, Policies, and Programs*. Vol. 1, Thousand Oaks, CA: Sage Publications.

Helms, J. E. and Cook, D. A. (1999). *UsingRace in Counseling and Psychotherapy: Theory and Process*, Needham, MA: Allyn & Bacon.

Helms, J.E. and Piper, R.E. (1994) 'Implications of racial identity theory for vocational psychology', *Journal of Vocational Behaviour*, 44:124–38.

Hemsley, G. D. and Doob, A. N. (1978) 'The effect of looking behavior on perceptions of a communicator's credibility', *Journal of Applied Social Psychology*, 8, 2: 136–44.

Hendricks, M. and Bootzin, R. (1976) 'Race and sex as stimuli for negative affect and physical avoidance', *Journal of Social Psychology*, 98: 111–20.

Henley, N. M. (1977) *Body Politics: Power, Sex, and Nonverbal Communication*, Englewood Cliffs, NJ: Prentice-Hall.

Henshall, C. and McGuire, J. (1986) 'Gender relations', in M. Richards and P. Light (eds.) *Children of Social Worlds*, Cambridge: Polity Press.

Hepworth, D. H. and Larsen, J. A. (1990) *Direct Social Work Practice: Theory and Skills*, Belmont, CA: Wadsworth.

Herbert, M. (1986) *Psychology for Social Workers*, London: Macmillan.

Hernstein, R. and Murray, C. (1994) *The Bell Curve: Intelligence and Class Structure in American Life*, New York: Free Press.

Hewitt, R. (1986) *White Talk Black Talk: Inter-Racial Friendship and Communication Among Adolescents*, Cambridge: Cambridge University Press.

Highlen, P. S. and Hill, C. E. (1984) 'Factors affecting client change in individual counseling: current status of theoretical speculations', in S. D. Brown and R. W. Lent (eds.) *The Handbook of Counseling Psychology*, New York: Harper & Row.

Hill, R. (1972) *Strengths of the Black Family*, New York: National Urban League.

Hill, R. (1977) *Informal Adoption Among Black Families*, Washington, DC: National Urban League.

Hill, R. (1999) *Strengths of the Black Family*, 2nd edn, New York: National Urban League.

Hill, R. (2003) *The Strengths of Black Families*, 2nd edn, Lanham, MD: University Press of America.

Hill, S. A. (1998) *African American Children: Socialization and Development in Families*, Thousand Oaks, CA: Sage Publications.

Hilliard, A. G. (1981) 'IQ thinking as catechism: ethnic and cultural bias or invalid science', *Black Books Bulletin*, 17, 2: 2–7.

Hilliard, A. G. (1987) 'The ideology of intelligence and IQ magic in education', *The Negro Educational Review*, 38, 2: 136–45.

Hilliard, A. G. (2004) 'Intelligence: What good is it and why bother to measure it?', in R. L. Jones (ed.) *Black Psychology*, 4th edn, Berkeley, CA: Cobb & Henry.

Hines, P.M., Garcia-Preto, N., McGoldrick, M., Almeida, R., and Weltman, S. (1992) 'Intergenerational relationships across cultures', *The Journal of Contemporary Human Services*, 23: 323–38.

Hinton, P. (1993) *The Psychology of Interpersonal Perception*, London: Routledge.

Hinton, P. (2000) *The Psychology of Interpersonal Perception*, London: Routledge.

Hitch, P.J. (1981) 'Immigration and mental health: local research and social explanations', *New Community* 9, 2: 256–62.

Hitch, P. and Clegg, P. (1980) 'Modes of referral of overseas immigrant and native born first admissions to psychiatric hospital', *Social Science and Medicine*, 11: 369–74.

Holdstock, L. (2001) *Re-Examining Psychology: Critical Perspectives and African Insights*, London: Routledge.

Hooks, B. (1984) *Ain't I a Woman: Black Women and Feminism*, London: Pluto Press.

Hraba, J. and Grant, G. (1970) 'Black is beautiful: a re-examination of racial preference and identification', *Journal of Personality and Social Psychology*, 16: 398–402.

Hunt, J. M. (1961) *Intelligence and Experience*, New York: Ronald Press.

Hurdle, D. (1990) 'The ethnic group experience', in K.L. Chau (ed.) *Ethnicity and Biculturalism: Emerging Perspectives of Social Group Work*, New York: Haworth Press.

Hutnik, N. (1991) *Ethnic Minority Identity: A Social Psychological Perspective*, Oxford: Oxford University Press.

Hylton, C. (1997) *Family Survival Strategies: Moyenda Black Families Talking*, London: Joseph Rowntree Foundation.

Ickes, W. (1984) 'Compositions in black and white: determinants of interaction in interracial dyads', *Journal of Personality and Social Psychology*, 47, 2: 330–41.

Ilahi, N. (1988) 'Psychotherapy services to the ethnic communities', report of a study in Ealing, London, unpublished paper.

Ince, L. (1998) *Making it Alone: A Study of the Care Experiences of Young Black People*, London: BAAF.

Ineichen, B. (1984) 'Mental illness among New Commonwealth migrants', in A. J. Bower (ed.) *Mobility and Migration: Biosocial Aspects of Human Movement*, London: Taylor & Francis.

Irvine, J. J. (1990) *Black Students and School Failure; Policies, Practices and Perceptions*, New York: Greenwood.

Jackson, B. (1975) 'Black identity development', in L. Golubschick and B. Persky (eds.) *Urban Social and Educational Issues*, Dubuque, IA: Kendall/Hunt.

Jackson, G. (1976) 'The African genesis of the Black perspective in helping', *Professional Psychology*, 7, 3: 292–308.

Jackson, G. G. (1979) 'The origin and development of black psychology: implications for black studies and human behaviour', *Studia Africana*, 1, 3: 270–93.

Jackson-Lowman, H. (2004) 'Perspectives on Afrikan American mental health: Lessons from Afrikan systems', in R. L. Jones (ed.) *Black Psychology*, 4th edn, Berkeley, CA: Cobb & Henry.

Jacobs, J. H. (1992) 'Identity development in biracial children', in M. P. Root (ed.) *Racially Mixed People in America*, Newbury Park, CA: Sage Publications.

Jahoda, G., Dasen, P. R. (1986) 'A cross-cultural perspective on developmental psychology', *International Journal of Behavioural Development*, 9: 417–37.

Jenkins, A. H. (1982) *The Psychology of the Afro-American: A Humanistic Approach*, Elmsford, NY: Pergamon.

Jensen, A. (1969) 'How much can we boost I.Q. and scholastic achievement?', *Harvard Educational Review*, 39: 1–23.

Jensen, A. R. (1987) 'Further evidence for Spearman's hypothesis concerning black-white differences on psychometric tests', *Behavioral and Brain Sciences*, 10: 512–19.

Johnson, K. R. (1971) 'Black kinesics: some nonverbal communication patterns in black culture', *Florida Foreign Language Reporter*, 9: 17–20.

Johnson, F. L. and Buttny, R. (1982) 'White listeners' responses to "sounding Black" and "sounding White": the effects of message content on judgements about language', *Communication Monographs*, 49: 33–49.

Johnson, D. J., Jaeger, E., Randolph, S. M., Cauce, A. M. and Ward, J. (2003) 'Studying the effects of early child care experiences on the development of children of color in the United States: Towards a more inclusive research agenda', *Child Development*, 74, 5: 1227–44.

Jones, R. (1999) *Teaching Racism – or Tackling It? Multicultural stories from white beginning teachers*, Stoke on Trent: Trentham Books.

Jones, R.L. (1991) *Black Psychology*, 3rd edn, Berkeley, CA: Cobb & Henry.

Jones, R. L. (2004) (ed.) *Black Psychology*, 4th edn, Berkeley, CA: Cobb & Henry.

Jones, E. E. and Korchin, S. J. (eds.) (1982) *Minority Mental Health*, New York: Praeger.

Jones, M. and Jones, M. (1970) 'The neglected client', *Black Scholar*, 1: 35–42.

Jordan, T. J. (1981) 'Self-concept, motivation and academic achievement of black adolescents', *Journal of Educational Psychology*, 73, 4: 509–17.

Joseph, G., Reddy, V. and Searle-Chatterjee, M. (1990) 'Eurocentrism, in the social sciences', *Race and Class*, 31, 4: 1–26.

Jung, C. (1950) 'On the psychology of the Negro', in W. McGuire (ed.) *Collected Works of Carl G. Jung*, Vol. 18, Princeton, NJ: Princeton University Press.

Kadushin, A. (1990) *The Social Work Interview*, New York: Columbia University Press.

Kadushin, A. (1997) *The Social Work Interview*, 2nd edn, New York: Columbia University Press.

Kallgren, C. A. and Caudill, P. J. (1993) 'Current transracial adoption practices: racial dissonance or racial awareness', *Psychological Reports* 72, 2: 551–8.

Kambon, K. K. (1992) *The African Personality in America: An African-centered Framework*, Tallahassee, FL: Nubian Nation Publications.

Kambon, K. K. (1998) *African/Black Psychology in the American Context: An African-centred Approach*, Tallahassee, FL: Nubian Nation Publications.

Kambon, K. K. (2004) 'The worldviews paradigms as the conceptual framework for African/Black psychology' in R. L. Jones (ed.) *Black Psychology*, 4th edn, Berkeley, CA: Cobb & Henry.

Kardiner, A. and Ovessey, L. (1951) *The Mark of Oppression*, New York: Norton.

Kareem, J. (1988) 'Outside in, inside out: some considerations in intercultural psychotherapy', *Journal of Social Work Practice*, 3, 3: 57–71.

Kareem, J. (1993) 'Outside in, inside out: some considerations in intercultural psycho-therapy', in P. Clarke, M. Harrison, K. Patel, M. Shah, M. Varley and T. Zack-Williams, *Improving Mental Health Practice*, Leeds: CCETSW.

Kareem. J. and Littlewood. R. (1999) *Intercultural Therapy – Themes. Interpretations and Practice*, 2nd edn, Oxford: Blackwell Scientific Publications.

Karenga, M. (1982) *Introduction to Black Studies*, Inglewood, CA: Kawaida Publications.

Katz, J. H. (1985) 'The socio-political nature of counseling', *The Counseling Psychologist*, 13: 615–24.

Katz, I. and Benjamin, L. (1960) 'Effects of white authoritarianism in biracial work groups', *Journal of Abnormal and Social Psychology*, 61: 448–56.

Katz, I. and Greenbaum, C. (1963) 'Effects of anxiety, threat, and racial environment on task performance of Negro college students', *Journal of Abnormal and Social Psychology*, 66: 562–7.

Katz, J. H. and Ivey, A. (1977) 'White awareness: the frontier of racism awareness training', *The Personnel and Guidance Journal*, 55: 485–9.

Kaye, C. and Lingiah, T. (2000) *Race, culture and ethnicity in secure psychiatric practice; Working with difference*, London: Jessica Kingsley Publishers.

Keating, F., Robertson, D., McCulloch, A. and Francis, E. (2002) *Breaking the Circles of Fear*, London: Sainsbury Centre for Mental Health.

Kelly, A. (1988) 'Ethnic differences in science choice, attitudes and achievement in Britain', *British Educational Research Journal*, 14, 2: 113–20.

Kempadoo, M. and Abdelrazak, M. (2001) *Directory of Supplementary and Mother-tongue Classes*, London: Resource Unit.

Kendon, A. (1967) 'Some functions of gaze direction in social interaction', *Acta Psychologica*, 71: 359–72.

Kerwin, C. and Ponterotto, J. G. (1995) 'Biracial identity development: Theory and research', in J. G. Ponterotto, J. M. Casas, L. A. Suzuki and C. M. Alexander (eds.) *Handbook of Multicultural Counseling*, Thousand Oaks, CA: Sage Publications.

Khan, A. (1983) 'The mental health of the Asian community in an East London health district', in *Care in the Community: Keeping It Local*, report of MIND annual conference.

Khan, V. (ed.) (1979) *Minority Families in Britain*, London: Macmillan.

Khatib, S. M., Akbar, N., McGee, D. P. and Nobles, W. (1975) 'Voodoo or IQ: an introduction to African psychology', *Journal of Black Psychology*, 1, 2: 9–29.

Kibria, N. (1997) 'The construction of 'Asian American': Reflections on intermarriage and ethnic identity among second generation Chinese and Korean Americans', *Ethnic and Racial Studies*, 20: 523–44.

Kincaid, M. (1968) 'Identity and therapy in the black community', *Personnel and Guidance Journal*, 47: 884–90.

King, N. G. and James, M. J. (1983) 'The relevance of black English to intercultural communication', paper presented at the *Annual Conference of the Western Speech Communication Association*, Albuquerque, NM.

Kleinke, C. L. (1986) 'Gaze and eye contact: a research review', *Psychological Bulletin*, 100, 1: 78–100.

Knapp, M. L. (1972) 'The field of nonverbal communication: an overview', in C. J. Stewart and B. Kendall (eds.) *On Speech Communication: An Anthology of Contemporary Writings and Messages*, New York: Holt, Rinehart & Winston.

Knapp, M. L. (1978) *Nonverbal Communication in Human Interaction*, New York: Holt, Rinehart & Winston.

Knapp, M. L. (1980) *Essentials of Nonverbal Communication*, New York: Holt, Rinehart & Winston.

Knapp, M. and Hall, J. (2006). *Nonverbal Communication in Human Interaction*, 6th edn, Belmont, CA: Thomson Wadsworth.

Konopka, G. (1983) *Social Group Work: A Helping Process*, Englewood Cliffs, NJ: Prentice-Hall.

Korchin, S. J. (1980) 'Clinical psychology and minority problems', *American Psychologist*, 35, 3: 262–9.

Kraut, R. E. and Poe, D. (1980) 'On the line: the deception judgements of custom inspectors and laymen', *Journal of Personality and Social Psychology*, 36: 380–91.

Kunjufu, J. (1985) *Countering the Conspiracy to Destroy Black Boys*, Vol. 2, Chicago, IL: African American Images.

Labov, W. P. (1982) 'Objectivity and commitment in linguistic science: the case of the Black English trial in Ann Arbor', *Language in Society*, 11: 165–201.

Ladner, J. (1971) *Tomorrow's Tomorrow: The Black Woman*, Garden City, NY: Doubleday.

LaFrance, M. and Mayo, C. (1976) 'Racial differences in gaze behaviour during conversation: two systematic observational studies', *Journal of Personality and Social Psychology*, 33: 547–52.

Lashley, H. and Pumfrey, P. (1993) 'Countering racism in British education', in G. K. Verma and P. D. Pumfrey (eds.) *Cross Curricular Contexts: Themes and Dimensions in Secondary Schools*, London: Falmer Press.

Lau, A. (1988) 'Family therapy and ethnic minorities', in E. Street and W. Dryden (eds.) *Family Therapy in Britain*, Milton Keynes: Open University Press.

Lau, A. (2002) 'Family therapy and ethnic minorities', in K. N. Dwivedi (ed.) *Meeting the Needs of Ethnic Minority Children: Including Refugee, Black, and Mixed Parentage Children: A Handbook for Professionals*, London, Jessica Kingsley Publishers.

Lawrence, E. (1982) 'In the abundance of water: the fool is thirsty', in Centre for Contemporary Cultural Studies, *The Empire Strikes Back*, London: Hutchinson.

Leong, F. (1992) 'Guidelines for minimizing premature termination among Asian American clients in group counseling', *The Journal for Specialists in Group Work*, 17, 4: 218–28.

Lester, H. and Glasby, J. (2006) *Mental Health Policy and Practice*, London; Macmillan.

Lewis, D. K. and Looney, J. (1983) *The Long Struggle: Well-functioning Working Class Black Families*, New York: Brunner/Mazel.

Lewis, G., Croft-Jeffreys, C. and David, A. (1990) 'Are British psychiatrists racist?', *British Journal of Psychiatry*, 157: 411–15.

Liebkind, K. and Jasinskaja-Lahti, I. (2000) 'Acculturation and psychological well-being among immigrant adolescents in Finland: A comparative study of adolescents from different cultural backgrounds', *Journal of Adolescent Research*, 15: 446–69.

Lippman, W. (1922) *Public Opinion*, New York: Harcourt, Brace.

Littlewood, R. (1988) 'Community-initiated research: a study of psychiatrists' conceptualizations of "cannabis psychosis"', *Psychiatric Bulletin*, 12: 486–8.

Littlewood, R. (1992) 'DSM-IV and culture: Is the classification intentionally valid?', *Psychiatric Bulletin*, 16: 257–61.

Littlewood, R. and Cross, S. (1980) 'Ethnic minorities and psychiatric services', *Sociology of Health and Illness*, 2, 2: 194–201.

Littlewood, R. and Lipsedge, M. (1981a) 'Some social and phenomenological characteristics of psychotic immigrants', *Psychological Medicine*, 11: 289–302.

Littlewood, R. and Lipsedge, M. (1981b) 'Acute psychotic reactions in Caribbean-born patients', *Psychological Medicine*, 11: 303–18.

Littlewood, R. and Lipsedge, M. (1997) *Aliens and Alienists: Ethnic Minorities and Psychiatry*, 3rd edn, London: Routledge.

Longino, H. E. (1990) *Science as Social Knowledge: Values and Objectivity in Scientific Inquiry*, Princeton, NJ: Princeton University Press.

Looney, J. (1988) 'Ego development and black identity', *The Journal of Black Psychology*, 15, 1: 41–56.

Lorde, A. (1984) *Sister Outsider*, New York: The Crossing Press.

Loring, M. and Powell, B. (1988) 'Gender, race and DSM-III: a study of the objectivity of psychiatric diagnostic behaviour', *Journal of Health and Social Behaviour*, 29: 1–22.

Louden, D. (1978) 'A comparative study of self-esteem and locus of control in minority group adolescents', unpublished PhD thesis, University of Bristol.

Luthra, M. (1997) *Britain's Black Population*, Aldershot: Arena.

Mabey, C. (1986) 'Black pupils' achievement in Inner London', *Educational Research*, 28, 3: 163–73.

McAdoo, H. P. (1978) *Black Youth*, Milton Keynes: Open University Press.

McAdoo, H. P. (1981a) *Black Families*, Beverly Hills, CA: Sage Publications.

McAdoo, H. P. (1981b) 'Upward mobility and parenting in middle-income black families', *Journal of Black Psychology*, 8, 1:1–22.

McAdoo, H. P. (1985) 'The development of self-concept and race attitudes of young black children over time', in *Black Families*, 2nd edn, London: Sage Publications.

McAdoo, H. P. (1988) 'Preface to the first edition', in *Black Families*, 2nd edn, London: Sage Publications.

McAdoo, H. P. (1992) 'The study of ethnic minority families: implications for practitioners and policy makers', in K. Adams (ed.) *Cultural Diversity in Families*, New York: Brown and Benchmark.

McAdoo, H. P. (1995) 'Stress levels, family help patterns and religiosity in middle and working class African American single mothers', *Journal of Black Psychology*, 21, 424–49.

McAdoo, H. P. (1996) *Black Families*, Thousand Oaks, CA: Sage Publications.

McAdoo, H. P. (1997) *Black Families*, 3rd edn, Thousand Oaks, CA: Sage Publications.

McAdoo, H. P. (1999) *Family Ethnicity: Strength in Diversity*, Thousand Oaks, CA: Sage Publications.

McAdoo, H. P. (ed.) (2002) *Black Children*, 2nd edn, Thousand Oaks, CA: Sage Publications.

McAdoo, H. P. and McAdoo, J. L. (eds.) (1985) *Black Children: Social, Educational and Parental Environments*, Beverly Hills, CA: Sage Publications.

McAdoo, J. L. (1979) 'Father-child interaction patterns and self-esteem in Black pre-school children', *Young Children*, 34, 1: 46–53.

Mac an Ghaill, M. (1988) *Young, Gifted and Black*, Buckingham: Open University Press

McAvoy, B. and Sayeed, A. (1994) 'Communication', in B. R. McAvoy and L. J. Donaldson (eds.) *Health Care for Asians*, Oxford: Oxford University Press.

McCarthy, J. and Yancey, W. L. (1971) 'Uncle Tom and Mr. Charlie: metaphysical pathos in the study of racism and personal disorganization', *American Journal of Sociology*, 76: 648–72.

McDougall, W. (1921) *Is America Safe for Democracy?*, New York: Scribner.

McGovern, D. and Cope, R. (1987) 'Compulsory detention of males of different ethnic groups with special reference to offender status', *British Journal of Psychiatry*, 150: 505–12.

McKenzie, K. (2003) 'Racism and health', *British Medical Journal*, 326: 880.

McKenzie, K., Samele, C., Van Horn, E., Tattan, T., Van Os, J., Murray, R. (2001) 'Comparison of the outcome and treatment of psychosis in people of Caribbean origin living in the UK and British Whites. Report from the UK700 trial', *The British Journal of Psychiatry*, 178: 160–5.

McLean, C., Campbell, C. and Cornish, F. (2003) 'African-Caribbean interactions with mental health services in the UK: experiences and expectations of exclusion as (re)productive of health inequalities', *Social Science and Medicine*, 56, 3: 657–69.

MacPherson, W. (1999) *The Stephen Lawrence Inquiry*, London: Stationery Office.

McRoy, R. G. and Zurcher, L. A. (1983) *Transracial and Inracial Adoptees*, Springfield, IL: Charles C. Thomas.

Madhere, S. (1995) 'Beyond the bell curve: Toward a model of talent and character development', *Journal of Negro Education*, 64(3): 326–39.

Majors, R. (1991) 'Nonverbal behaviors and communication styles among African Americans', in R. Jones (ed.) *Black Psychology*, 3rd edn, Berkeley, CA: Cobb & Henry.

Majors, R. (ed.) (2001) *Educating Our Black Children: New Directions and Radical Approaches*, London: Routledge.

Majors, R., Gillborn, S. and Sewell, T. (2001) 'The exclusion of black children: implications for a racialised perspective', in R. Majors (ed.) *Educating Our Black Children: New Directions and Radical Approaches*, London: Routledge.

Malcolm, X. (1965) *The Autobiography of Malcolm X*, New York: Grove Press.

Manusov, V. and Patterson, M.L. (2006) *The Sage Handbook of Non-verbal Communication*, Thousand Oaks, CA: Sage Publications.

Marshall, S. (1995) 'Ethnic socialization of African American children: Implications for parenting, identity development, and academic performance', *Journal of Youth and Adolescence*, 24, 4: 337–96.

Marks, B., Settles, I. H., Cooke, D. Y., Morgan, L. and Sellers, R. (2004) 'African American racial identity: A review of contemporary models and measures', in R. L. Jones (ed.) *Black Psychology*, 4th edn, Berkeley, CA: Cobb & Henry.

Martin, E. P. and Martin, J. M. (1978) *The Black Extended Family*, Chicago, IL: University of Chicago Press.

Mathias, A. (1978) 'Contrasting approaches to the study of black families', *Journal of Marriage and the Family*, 40: 667–76.

Matsumoto, D. (2001) *The Handbook of Culture and Psychology*, New York: Oxford University Press.

Matsumoto, D. (2006) Culture and nonverbal behaviour, in Manusov, V., Patterson, M. (eds.), *Handbook of Nonverbal Communication*, Thousand Oaks, CA: Sage Publications.

Matthews-Juarez, P. (1982) *The Effect of Family Backgrounds on the Educational Outcome of Black Teenagers in Worcester, Massachusetts*, Ann Arbor, MI: University Microfilms International.

Maultsby, M. (1982) 'A historical view of Blacks' distrust of psychiatry', in S. M. Turner and R. T. Jones (eds.) *Behaviour Modification in Black Populations*, New York: Plenum.

Maxime, J. (1986) 'Some psychological models of black self-concept', in S. Ahmed, J. Cheetham, and J. Small (eds.) *Social Work with Children and their Families*, London: Batsford.

Maxime, J. (1987) *Black Like Me – Workbook One: Black Identity*, Kent: Emani Publications.

Maxime, J. (1991) *Black Like Me – Workbook Two: Black Pioneers*, Kent: Emani Publications.

Maxime, J. (1993) 'The therapeutic importance of racial identity in working with Black children who hate', in V. Varma (ed.) *How and Why Children Hate*, London: Jessica Kingsley Publishers.

Maxime, J. (1997) 'Some psychological models of black self-concept', in S. Ahmed, J. Cheetham, and J. Small (eds.) *Social Work with Children and their Families*, 2nd edn, London: Batsford.

Mead, G. (1934) 'Mind, self and society', in A. Strauss (ed.) *George Herbert Mead: On Social Psychology*, Chicago, IL: University of Chicago Press.

Mehrabian, A. and Ferris, S. R. (1967) 'Inference of attitudes from nonverbal communication in two channels', *Journal of Consulting Psychology*, 31: 248–52.

Mercer, K. (1984) 'Black communities' experience of psychiatric services', *International Journal of Social Psychiatry*, 30: 22–7.

Mercer, K. (1993) 'Racism and transcultural psychiatry', in P. Clarke, M. Harrison, K. Patel, M. Shah, M. Varley and T. Zack-Williams, *Improving Mental Health Practice*, Leeds: CCETSW.

Miller, D. (1985) 'Proud to be black', *Community Care*, 21 February: 18–19.

Milliones, J. (1973) 'Construction of the developmental inventory of black consciousness', PhD thesis, University of Pittsburgh.

Milner, D. (1975) *Children and Race*, Harmondsworth: Penguin.

Milner, D. (1982) 'The education of the black child in Britain: a review and response', *New Community*, 9, 2: 289–93.

Milner, D. (1983) *Children and Race: Ten Years On*, London: Ward Lock Educational.

Mirza, H. (1992) *Young, Female and Black*, London: Routledge.

Mirza, H. and Reay, D. (2000) 'Spaces and places of black educational desire: Rethinking black supplementary schools as a new social movement, *Sociology*, 34, 3: 521–44.

Mitchell, H. and Lewter, N. (1986) *Soul Theology: The Heart of American Black Culture*, San Francisco, CA: Harper & Row.

Modood, T. (2003) 'Ethnic differences in educational attainment', in D. Mason (ed.) *Explaining Ethnic Differences*, Bristol: Policy Press.

Modood, T. (2005) *Multicultural Politics: Racism, Ethnicity and Muslims in Britain*, Minneapolis, MN and Edinburgh: University of Minnesota Press.

Modood, T., Berthoud, R. and Virdee, S. (1994) *Changing Ethnic Identities*, London Policy Studies Institute.

Modood, T., Berthoud, R., Lakey, J., Nazroo, J., Smith, P., Virdee, S. and Beishon, S. (1997) *Ethnic Minorities in Britain: Diversity and Disadvantage*, London, Policy Studies Institute.

Moreno, J. L. (1934) *Who shall Survive?* Washington, DC: Nerrow & Mental, No. 58.

Morgan, C., Mallett, R., Hutchinson, G., Bagalkote, H., Morgan, K., Fearon, P., Dazzan, P., Boydell, J., Harrison, G., Murray, R., Jones, P., Craig, T., and Leff, J. on behalf of the ÆSOP Study Group (2005) 'Pathways To Care And Ethnicity I. Sample Characteristics And Compulsory Admission – A Report From The Æsop (Aetiology And Ethnicity In Schizophrenia And Other Psychoses) Study', *British Journal of Psychiatry*, 186: 281–9

Morgan, H. (1995) *Historical Perspectives on the Education of Black Children*, Westport, CT: Praeger.

Morland, J. K. (1958) 'Racial recognition by nursery school children in Lynchburg, Virginia', *Social Forces*, 37: 132–7.

Mosby, D. P. (1972) 'Toward a new speciality of black psychology', in R. Jones (ed.) *Black Psychology*, New York: Harper & Row.

Moynihan, D. (1965) *The Negro Family: The Case for National Action*, Washington, DC: Office of Policy Planning and Research, US Department of Labour.

Mullender, A. (1990) 'The Ebony project – bicultural group work with transracial foster parents', *Social Work with Groups*, 13: 23–41.

Mullender, A. and Miller, D. (1985) 'The Ebony group: black children in white foster homes', *Adoption and Fostering*, 9, 1: 33–40.

Mullender, A. and Ward, D. (1985) 'Towards an alternative model of social group work', *British Journal of Social Work*, 15: 155–72.

Mullender, A. and Ward, D. (1991) *Self-Directed Groupwork: Users Take Action for Empowerment*, London: Whiting and Birch.

Murray, C. B. and Fairchild, H. (1989) 'Models of black adolescent academic underachievement', in R. Jones, *Black Adolescents*, Berkeley, CA: Cobb & Henry.

Murray, H. A. (1938) *Explorations in Personality*, New York: Oxford University Press.

Mussen, P. H., Conger, J. J., Kagan, J. and Huston, A. C. (1984) *Child Development and Personality*, New York: Harper & Row.

Myers, H. F. (1982) 'Research on the Afro-American family: a critical review', in B. Bass, G. E. Wyatt and G. Powell (eds.) *The Afro-American Family: Assessment, Treatment and Research*, New York: Grune & Stratton.

Myers, H. I. and King, L. M. (1980) 'Youth of the Black underclass: Urban stress and mental health', *Fanon Centre Journal*, 1:1–27.

Myers, L. (1988) *Understanding an Afrocentric World View: Introduction to an Optimal Psychology*, Dubuque, IA: Kendall/Hunt.

Myes, H. J. and Yochelson, L. (1949) 'Color denial in the Negro', *Psychiatry*, 11: 39–42.

Ndetei, D. M. (1986) 'Paranoid disorder: environmental, cultural or constitutional phenomenon', *Acta Psychiatrica Scandinavica*, 74: 50–4.

Nickerson, K. J., Helms, J. E. and Terrell, F. (1994) 'Cultural mistrust, opinions about mental illness, and Black students' attitudes toward seeking psychological help from White counselors', *Journal of Counseling Psychology*, 41, 3: 378–85.

Nicolson, P. and Bayne, R. (1984) *Applied Psychology for Social Workers*, London: Macmillan.

Nicolson, P. and Bayne, R. (1990) *Applied Psychology for Social Workers*, 2nd edn, London: Macmillan.

Nicolson, P., Bayne, R. and Owen, J. (1990) *Applied Psychology for Social Workers*, 2nd edn, London: Macmillan.

Nicolson, P., Bayne, R. and Owen, J. (2006) *Applied Psychology for Social Workers*, 3rd edn, London: Macmillan.

Nobles, W. (1972) 'African philosophy: foundations for black psychology', in R. Jones (ed.) *Black Psychology*, New York: Harper & Row.

Nobles, W. (1973) 'Psychological research and the Black self concept: a critical review', *Journal of Social Issues*, 29, 1: 11–31.

Nobles, W. (1974) 'African root and American fruit: the black family', *Journal of Social and Behavioral Sciences*, 20: 52–64.

Nobles, W. (1976) 'Black people in white insanity: an issue for black community mental health', *Journal of Afro-American Issues*, 4: 21–7.

Nobles, W. (1978) 'Toward an empirical and theoretical framework for defining black families', *Journal of Marriage and Family*, November: 679–88.

Nobles, W. (1980) 'African philosophy: foundations for black psychology', in R. Jones (ed.) *Black Psychology*, 2nd edn, New York: Harper & Row.

Nobles, W. (1986) *African Psychology*, Oakland, CA: Black Family Institute.

Nobles, W. (2004) 'African philosophy: Foundations for Black psychology', in R. Jones (ed.) *Black Psychology*, 4th edn, New York: Harper & Row.

Norton, D. G. (1983) 'Black family life patterns, the developments of self and cognitive development of Black children', in G. Powell, J. Yamamoto and E. Morales (eds.) *The Psychosocial Development of Minority Group Children*, New York: Brunner/Mazel.

Nsamenang, A. B. (1995) 'Theories of developmental psychology for a cultural perspective: A view from Africa', *Psychology and Developing Societies*, 7: 1–19.

NSPCC (1999) *Protecting Children from Racism and Racial Abuse, A Research Review*, London: NSPCC.

OfSTED (1999) *Raising the Attainment of Minority Ethnic Pupils: School and LEA's Response*, London: OfSTED.

O'Neale, V. (2000) *Excellence not Excuses: Inspection of Services for Ethnic Minority Children and Families*, London: Social Services Inspectorate.

Onwubu, C. (1990) 'The intellectual foundations of racism', in T. Anderson (ed.) *Black Studies: Theory, Method and Cultural Perspectives*, Pullman, WA: Washington State University Press.

Onyango, R. S. (1986) 'Cannabis psychosis in young psychiatric inpatients', *British Journal of Addiction*, 81: 419–23.

Osborne, J. W. (2001). 'Academic disidentification: Unraveling underachievement among Black boys', in R. Majors (ed.) *Educating Our Black Children: New Directions and Radical Approaches*, London: Routledge.

Padilla, A. M. and Ruiz, R. A. (1975) 'Personality assessment and test interpretation of Mexican-Americans: a critique', *Journal of Personality Assessment*, 39: 103–9.

Palardy, J. M. (1969) 'What teachers believe – what children achieve', *Elementary School Journal*, 69: 370–4.

Parekh, B. (1983) 'Educational opportunity in multi-ethnic Britain', in N. Glazer and K. Young (eds.) *Ethnic Pluralism and Public Policy*, London: Heinemann.

Parekh, B. (1986) 'The concept of multicultural education', in S. Mogdil, G. K.Verma, K. Mallick, and C. Modgil (eds.) *Multicultural Education: The Interminable Debate*, Lewes: Falmer.

Parekh, B. (ed.) (2000) *The Future of Multiethnic Britain*, London: Profile Books.

Parham, T. A. (1989) 'Cycles of psychological nigrescence', *The Counseling Psychologist*, 17, 2: 187–226.

Parham, T. A. (2002) *Counseling Persons of African Descent*, Thousand Oaks, CA: Sage Publications.

Parham, T. A. and Helms, J. E. (1981) 'The influence of Black students' racial identity attitudes on preference for counselor's race', *Journal of Counseling Psychology*, 28: 250–7.

Parham, T. A. and Helms, J. E. (1985) 'Relation of racial identity to self-actualization and affective states of black students', *Journal of Counseling Psychology*, 28, 3: 250–6.

Parham, T. A. and Williams, P. T. (1993) 'The relationship of demographic and background factors to racial identity attitudes', *Journal of Black Psychology*, 19, 1: 7–24.

Parham, T. A. and White, J. L. (1990) *The Psychology of Blacks: An African American Perspective*, Englewood Cliffs, NJ: Prentice-Hall.

Parmar, P. (1981) 'Young Asian women: a critique of the pathological approach', *Multi-Racial Education*, 9, 3: 19–29.

Penketh, L. (2000) *Tackling Institutional Racism: Anti-racist Policies and Social Work. Education and Training*, Bristol: Policy Press.

Pennie, P. and Best, F. (1990) *How the Black Family is Pathologised by the Social Services Systems*, London: ABSWAP.

Peters, M. F. (1976) 'Nine black families: a study of household management and childrearing in Black families with working mothers', PhD dissertation, Harvard University.

Peters, M. F. (1985) 'Racial socialization of young black children', in H. P. McAdoo and J. L. McAdoo (eds.) *Black Children*, Beverly Hills, CA: Sage Publications.

Peters, M. F. (1988) 'Parenting in black families with young children: a historical perspective', in H. P. McAdoo (ed.) *Black Families*, London: Sage Publications.

Pettigrew, T. (1964) *A Profile of the Negro American*, New York: Van Nostrand.

Phinney, J. S. (1989) 'Stages of ethnic identity development in minority group adolescents', *Journal of Early Adolescence*, 9: 34–49.

Phinney, J. S. (1990) 'Ethnic identity in adolescents and adults: Review of research', *Psychological Bulletin*, 108: 499–514.

Phinney, J.S. (1992) 'The multigroup ethnic identity measure: a new scale for use with diverse groups', *Journal of Adolescence*, 7, 2: 156–76

Phinney, J. S. (1999) 'An intercultural approach in psychology: cultural contact and identity', *Cross-Cultural Psychology Bulletin*, 33: 24–31.

Phinney, J. S. and Devich-Navarro, M. (1997) 'Variations in bicultural identification among African American and Mexican American adolescents', *Journal of Research on Adolescence*, 7: 3–32.

Phinney, J. S. and Kohatsu, E. L. (1997) 'Ethnic and racial identity development and mental health', in J. Schulenberg, J. Maggs and K. Hurrelman (eds.) *Health Risks and Developmental Transitions in Adolescence*, New York: Cambridge University Press.

Phoenix, A. (1988) 'The Afro-Caribbean Myth', *New Society* 4, March: 11–14.

Phoenix, A. (1990) 'Theories of gender and black families', in T. Lovell (ed.) *British Feminist Thought*, Oxford: Blackwell.

Phoenix, A. (1997) 'Theories of gender and black families', in H. Mirza (ed.) *Black British Feminism: A Reader*, London: Routledge.

Piaget, J. (1970) 'Piaget's theory', in P. Mussen (ed.) *Carmichael's Manual of Child Psychology*, Volume 1, New York: Wiley.

Pidgeon, D. A. (1970) *Expectations and Pupil Performance*, Slough: NFER.

Pinderhughes, E. (1995) 'Biracial identity: Asset or handicap?', in H. Harris, H. Blue and E. Griffiths (eds.) *Racial and Ethnic Identity*, London: Routledge.

Pinto, R. T. (1970) 'A study of psychiatric illness among Asians in the Camberwell area', MPhil dissertation, University of London.

Pipes, W. H. (1981) 'Old-time religion: benches can't say "Amen"', in H. McAdoo (ed.) *Black Families*, Beverley Hills, CA: Sage Publications.

Poortinga, Y. (1997) 'Towards convergence?', in J. W. Berry, Y. H. Poortinga and J. Pandey (eds.) *Handbook of Cross-Cultural Psychology*, Boston, MA: Allyn & Bacon.

Porter, J. R. and Washington, R. E. (1979) 'Black identity and self-esteem: a review of studies of black self-concept 1968–1978', *Annual Review of Sociology*, 5: 53–74.

Poston, W. S. C. (1990) 'The biracial identity development model: A needed addition', *Journal of Counseling and Development*, 69: 152–5.

Pouissant, A. (1974) 'Building a strong self-image in Black children', *Ebony Magazine* August: 138–43.

Powell, G. J. (1982) 'A six-city study of school desegregation and self-concept among Afro-American Junior High School students: a preliminary study with implications for mental health', in B. Bass, G. Wyatt and G. J. Powell (eds.) *The Afro-American Family, Assessment, Treatment and Research Issues*, New York: Grune & Stratton.

Powell, G. J. (1983) 'Self-concept in White and Black children', in C. V. Willie, B. M. Kramer and B. S. Brown (eds.) *Racism and Mental Health*, Pittsburgh: University of Pittsburgh.

Powell, G. J. and Fuller, M. (1970) 'Self-concept and school desegregation', *American Journal of Orthopsychiatry*, 40: 303.

Powell-Hopson, D. (1985) 'The effects of modeling, reinforcement, and color meaning word associations on doll color preferences of Black preschool children and White preschool children', unpublished doctoral dissertation, Hofstra University.

Powell-Hopson, D. and Hopson, D. S. (1990) *Different and Wonderful: Raising Black Children in a Race-conscious Society*, New York: Prentice-Hall.

Poyatos, F. (1992) *Paralanguage: Linguisitic and Interdisciplinary Approach to Speech and Interactive Sounds*, Amsterdam, Philadelphia, PA: John Benjamin.

Prevatt-Goldstein, B. and Spencer, M. (2000) *'Race' and Ethnicity*, London: British Agencies for Adoption and Fostering.

Proshansky, H. and Newton, P. (1968) 'The nature and meaning of Negro self-identity', in M. Deutsch, I. and A. R. Jensen (eds.) *Social Class, Race and Psychological Development*, New York: Holt, Rinehart & Winston.

Pugh, R. (1972) *Psychology of the Black Experience*, Belmont, CA: Wadsworth.

Rabiee, F. and Smith, P. (2007) *Being respected: An evaluation of the statutory and voluntary mental health service provision for members of African and African Caribbean communities in Birmingham*, Birmingham: University of Central England.

Rainwater, L. (1970) *Behind Ghetto Walls: Black Family Life in a Federal Slum*, Chicago, IL: Aldine.

Raleigh, V. S. (2000) 'Mental Health in Black and Ethnic Minorities: An Epidemiological Perspective', in Kaye, C. and Lingiah, T. (eds.) *Race, Culture and Ethnicity in Secure Psychiatric Practice: Working with Difference*, London: Jessica Kingsley Publishers.

Ramseur, H. P (2004) 'Psychologically healthy African American adults', in R. Jones (ed.) *Black Psychology*, 4th edn, Berkeley, CA: Cobb & Henry.

Raspberry, W. (1991) 'Right strategies for wrong countries', *New York Daily News*.

Reynolds, T. (1998) Afro-Caribbean mothering: Reconstructing a new identity, South Bank University, Unpublished PhD thesis.

Reynolds, T. (2000) 'Parenting, motherhood and paid work: Rationalities and ambivalences', London: ESRC Seminar series.

Ridley, C. (1995) *Overcoming Unintentional Racism in Counseling and Therapy: A Practitioner's Guide to Intentional Intervention*, Thousand Oaks, CA: Sage Publications.

Ridley, C. (2005) *Overcoming Unintentional Racism in Counseling and Therapy: A Practitioner's Guide to Intentional Intervention*, 2nd edn, Thousand Oaks, CA: Sage Publications.

Ringel, S. (2005) 'Group work with Asian American immigrants: A cross-cultural perspective', in model' in G. R. Grief and P. H. Ephross (2005) *Group Work with Populations at Risk*, Oxford: Oxford University Press.

Robinson, L. (1998) *Race, Communication and the Caring Professions*, Milton Keynes: Open University Press.

Robinson, L. (2000) 'Racial identity attitudes and self-esteem of black adolescents in residential care: An exploratory study', *British Journal of Social Work*, 30: 3–24.

Robinson, L. (2001) 'A conceptual framework for social work practice with black children and adolescents in the United Kingdom', *Journal of Social Work*, 1, 2: 165–85.

Robinson, L. (2003) 'The adaptation of Asian and African Caribbean second generation youth in Britain', Paper presented at the International Conference on Diversity in Organisations, Communications and Nations in Hawaii, 13–16 February.

Robinson, L. (2007) *Cross-cultural Child Development for Social Workers*, Basingstoke: Macmillan Press.

Rodriguez, R. F. and Lopez, L. C. (2003) 'Mexican-American parental involvement with a Texas elementary school', *Psychology Reports*, 92, 3: 791–2.

Root, M. P. (ed.) (1992) *Racially Mixed People in America*, Newbury Park, CA: Sage Publications.

Root, M. P. (ed.) (1996) *The Multiracial Experience: Racial Disorders as the New Frontier*, Thousand Oaks, CA: Sage Publications.

Rorschach, H. (1942) *Psychodiagnostics*, Berne: Huber.

Rosaldo, R. (1989) *Culture and Truth: The Remaking of Social Analysis*, Boston, MA: Beacon.

Rosenberg, M. (1979) *Conceiving the Self*, New York: Basic Books.

Rosenthal, R. and Jacobson, L. (1968) *Pygmalion in the Classroom*, New York: Holt, Rinehart & Winston.

Rotherdam, M. J. and Phinney, J.S. (1990) 'Patterns of social experiments among Black and Mexican-American children', *Child Development*, 61: 542–56

Rozelle, R. M. and Baxter, J. C. (1975) 'Impression formation and danger recognition in experienced police officers', *Journal of Social Psychology*, 96: 53–63.

Rubovitz, P. C. and Maehr, M. L. (1973) 'Pygmalion black and white', *Journal of Personality and Social Psychology*, 25, 2: 210–18.

Rushton, J. P. (1988a) 'Race differences in behaviour: a review and evolutionary analysis', *Personality and Individual Differences*, 9: 1009–24.

Rushton, J. P. (1988b) 'The reality of racial differences: a rejoinder with new evidence', *Personality and Individual Differences*, 9: 1035–40.

Ryan, W. (1967) 'Savage discovery: The Moynihan Report', in L. Rainwater and W. Yancey (eds.) *The Moynihan Report and the Politics of Controversy*, Cambridge, MA: MIT Press.

Ryan, W. (1971) *Blaming the Victim*, New York: Random House.

Samovar, L. A. and Porter, R. E. (2001) *Communication Between Cultures*, 4th edn, Belmont, CA: Wadsworth/Thomson Learning.

Samovar, L. and Porter, R. E. (2005) *Communication Between Cultures*, 6th edn, Belmont, CA: Wadsworth/Thomson Learning.

Samovar, L. A. and Porter, R. E. (2006) *Intercultural Communication: A Reader*, 11th edn, Belmont, CA: Wadsworth.

Samuda, R. J. (1975) *Psychological Testing of American Minorities*, New York: Harper & Row.

Sanches-Hucles, J. and Jones, N. (2005) 'Breaking the silence around race in training, practice and research', *The Counseling Psychologist*, 33, 4: 547–58.

Sanders Thompson, V. L. (1994) 'Socialization to race and its relationship to racial identification among African Americans', *Journal of Black Psychology*, 20, 2: 175–88.

Sashidaran, S. (1993) 'Schizophrenic or just black?', in P. Clarke, N. Patel, D. Naik, B. Humphries (eds.) *Improving Mental Health Practice*, Leeds: CCETSW.

Sashidharan, S. (2003) *Inside Outside: Improving Mental Health Services for Black and Minority Ethnic Communities in England*, London: National Institute for Mental Health in England.

Sattler, J. (1973) 'Racial experimenter effects', in K. S. Miller and R. M. Dreger (eds.) *Comparative Studies of Blacks and Whites in the United States*, New York: Seminar Press.

Sattler, J. (1977) 'The effects of therapist/client similarity', in A. Gurman and A. Razin (eds.) *Effective Psychotherapy: A Handbook of Research*, New York: Pergamon Press.

Scanzoni, J. (1971) *The Black Family in Modern Society*, Boston, MA: Allyn & Bacon.

Sebring, D. L. (1985) 'Considerations in counseling interracial children', *Journal of Non-White Concerns in Personnel and Guidance*, 13: 3–9.

Segal, L. (ed.) (1983) *What's To Be Done About The Family*, Harmondsworth: Penguin.

Segall, M. H., Dasen, P. R., Berry, J. W. and Poortinga, Y. H. (1990) *Human Behaviour in Global Perspective*, New York: Pergamon.

Segall, M. H., Lonner, W. J. and Berry, J. W. (1998) 'Cross cultural Psychology as a Scholarly Disciploine: On the Flowering of Culture in Behavioral Research', *American Psychologist*, 53, 10: 1101–10.

Semaj, L. T. (1980) 'The development of racial evaluation and preference: a cognitive approach', *Journal of Black Psychology*, 6, 2: 59–79.

Semaj, L. T. (1981) 'The black self', *Western Journal of Black Studies*, 5, 3: 158–71.

Seymour, H. N. and Seymour, C. M. (1979) 'The symbolism of ebonics: I'd rather switch than fight', *Journal of Black Studies*, 9: 397–410.

Shade, B. (1980) 'African American patterns of cognition', in R. Jones (ed.) *Black Psychology*, 2nd edn, New York: Harper & Row.

Shade, B. (1991) 'African American patterns of cognition', in R. Jones (ed.) *Black Psychology*, 3rd edn, New York: Harper & Row.

Shah, M. (1990) 'A study of Approved Social Workers' assessment of Black people under the Mental Health Act 1983', unpublished paper.

Shaikh, A. (1985) 'Cross-cultural comparison: psychiatric admissions of Asians and indigenous patients in Leicestershire', *International Journal of Social Psychiatry*, 31, 1: 3–11.

Shannon, B. (1973) 'The impact of racism on personality development', *Social Casework*, 54: 519–25.

Shaw, M. E. (1981) *Group Dynamics: The Psychology of Small Group Behaviour*, 3rd edn, New York: McGraw-Hill.

Shaw, A. (1988) *A Pakistani Community in Britain*, London: Blackwell.

Shipp, P. L. (1983) 'Counseling Blacks: a group approach', *Personnel and Guidance Journal*, 62: 108–11.

Short, G. (1985) 'Teacher expectations and West Indian under achievement', *Educational Research*, 27, 2: 95–101.

Sinclair, R. and Hai, N. (2002) *Children of Mixed Heritage in Need in Islington*, London: National Children's Bureau.

Singh, G. (1992) *Race and Social Work from 'Black Pathology' to 'Black Perspectives'*, Bradford: The Race Relations Unit.

Sinha, D. (1983) 'Cross-cultural psychology: a view from the Third World', in J. B. Deregowski, S. Dziurawier and R. C. Annis (eds.) *Explorations in Cross-Cultural Psychology*, Lisse: Swets & Zeitlinger.

Skellington, R. and Morris, P. (1992) *'Race' in Britain Today*, London: Open University.

Small, J. W. (1984) 'The crisis in adoption', *International Journal of Social Psychiatry*, 30, 1/2: 129–42.

Small, J. (1986) 'Transracial placements: conflicts and contradictions', in S. Ahmed, J. Cheetham, and J. Small (eds.) *Social Work with Black Children and their Families*, London: Batsford.

Smith, A. (1983) 'Nonverbal communication among black female dyads: an assessment of intimacy, gender and race', *Journal of Social Issues*, 39: 55–67.

Smith, D. and Tomlinson, S. (1989) *The School Effect: A Study of Multiracial Comprehensives*, London: Policy Studies Institute.

Smith, D. E., Willis, E. N. and Grier, J. A. (1980) 'Success and interpersonal touch in a competitive setting', *Journal of Nonverbal Behaviour*, 5: 26–34.

Smith, E. (1977) 'Counseling black individuals: some strategies', *Personnel and Guidance Journal*, 55: 390–6.

Smith, W. (1979) 'Which way black psychologists: tradition, modification or verification-innovation', in W. D. Smith, K. H. Burlew, M. H. Mosley and W. Whitney (eds.) *Reflections on Black Psychology*, Washington, DC: University Press of America.

Smith, W. D., Burlew, K. H., Mosley, M. and Whitney, W. (1978) *Minority Issues in Mental Health*, Reading, MA: Addison-Wesley.

Smith, W. D., Burlew, K. H., Mosley, M. and Whitney, W. (1979) *Reflections on Black Psychology*, Washington, DC: University Press of America.

Smitherman, G. (1977) *Talkin' and testifyin': The Language of Black America*, Boston, MA: Houghton Mifflin.

Smitherman, G. (2004) 'Talkin' and testifyin': Black English and the Black experience', in R. L. Jones (ed.) *Black Psychology*, 4th edn, Berkeley, CA: Cobb & Henry.

Smitherman, G. and McGinnis, J. (1972) 'Black language and Black liberation', in R. Jones (ed.) *Black Psychology*, New York: Harper & Row.

Smitherman-Donaldson, G. (1988) 'Discriminatory discourse on Afro-American speech', in G. Smitherman-Donaldson and T. A. Dijk (eds.) *Discourse and Discrimination*, Detroit, MI: Wayne State University Press.

Snowden, L. and Todman, P. (1982) 'The psychological assessment of blacks: new and needed developments', in E. E. Jones and S. J. Korchin (eds.) *Minority Mental Health*, New York: Praeger.

Sodowsky, G. R., Kwan, K. and Pannu, R. (1995) 'Ethnic identity of Asians in the United States: Conceptualizations and illustrations', in J. G. Ponterotto, J. M. Casas, L. A. Suzuki and C. M. Alexander (eds.) *Handbook of Multicultural Counseling*, Thousand Oaks, CA: Sage Publications.

Sondhi, R. (1982) 'The Asian Resource Centre – Birmingham', in A. Ohri, B. Manning, and P. Curno (eds.) *Community Work and Racism*, London: Routledge & Kegan Paul.

Spencer, M. B. (1982) 'Personal and group identity of Black children: an alternative synthesis', *Genetic Psychology Monographs*, 106: 59–84.

Spencer, M. B. (1983) 'Children's cultural values and parental child rearing strategies', *Developmental Review*, 3, 4: 351–70.

Spencer, M. B. (1984) 'Black children's race awareness, racial attitudes and self-concept: a reinterpretation', *Journal of Child Psychology and Psychiatry*, 25, 3: 433–41.

Spencer, M. B. (1988) 'Self concept development', in D. T. Slaughter (ed.) *Black Children in Poverty: Developmental Perspectives*, San Francisco, CA: Jossey-Bass.

Spencer, M. B., Nolls, E., Stoltzfus, J. and Harpalani, V. (2001) 'Identity and school adjustment: Revisiting the "Acting White" assumption', *Educational Psychologist*, 36, 1: 21–30.

Spencer, M. B. and Harpalani, V. (2006) 'What does "acting white" actually mean?', in J. Ogbu (ed.) *Minority Status, Collective Identity and Schooling*, Mahwan, NJ: Lawrence Erlbaum Associates.

Spencer, M. S., and Chen, J. (2004) 'Effect of discrimination on mental health service utilization among Chinese Americans', *American Journal Public Health*, May, 94, 5: 809–14.

Stack, C. (1974) *All Our Kin: Strategies for Survival in a Black Community*, New York: Harper & Row.

Staples, R. (ed.) (1971) *The Black Family: Essays and Studies*, Belmont, CA: Wadsworth.

Staples, R. (1974) 'The black family in evolutionary perspective', *Black Scholar* 5, 9: 2–9.

Staples, R. and Mirande, A. (1980) 'Racial and cultural variations among American families: an analytic review of the literature on minority families', *Journal of Marriage and the Family*, 42: 887–904.

Steele, C. M. and Aronson, J. (1995) 'Stereotype threat and the intellectual test performance of African Americans', *Journal of Personality and Social Psychology*, Nov 69, 5: 797–811.

Steele, C. M. and Aronson, J. (1998) 'Stereotype threat and the test performance of academically successful African Americans', in C. Jencks and M. Phillips (eds.) *The Black-White Test Score Group*, Washington: Brookings Institute.

Steele, R. E. and Davis, S. E. (1983) 'An empirical and theoretical review of articles in the *Journal of Black Psychology*: 1974–1980', *The Journal of Black Psychology*, 10, 1: 29–42.

Stephan, W. (1978) 'School desegregation: an evaluation of predictions made in Brown vs. Board of Education', *Psychological Bulletin*, 85: 217–38.

Stephan, C.W. (1992) 'Mixed heritage individuals: Ethnic identity and trait characteristics, in M. P. Root (ed.) *Racially Mixed People in America*, Newbury Park, CA: Sage Publications.

Stevenson, H. W. and Stewart, E. C. (1958) 'A developmental study of racial awareness in young children', *Child Development*, 29: 399–409.

Stevenson, H. (1994) 'Racial socialization in African American families: the art of balancing intolerance and survival', *The Family Journal: Counseling and Therapy for Couples and Families*, 2, 3: 190–8.

Stevenson, H. (1995) 'Relationship of adolescent perceptions of racial socialization to racial identity', *Journal of Black Psychology*, 21, 1: 49–70.

Stevenson, H. C. (1998) 'Theoretical considerations in measuring racial identity and socialization: Extending the self further', in R. L. Jones (ed.) *African American Identity Development*, Hampton, VA: Cobb & Henry.

Stevenson, H., Cameron, R., Herrero-Taylor, T. and Davis, G. (2002) 'Development of the Teenager Experience of Racial Socialization Scale: Correlates of Race-Related Socialization Frequency from the Perspective of Black Youth', *Journal of Black Psychology*, 28, 2: 84–106.

Stevenson, H. and Davis, G. (2004) 'Racial socialization', in Jones, R. L. (2004) (ed.) *Black Psychology*, 4th edn, Berkeley, CA: Cobb & Henry.

Stone, G. L. (ed.) (1990) 'Special issue on group therapy', *The Counseling Psychologist*, 18: 5–131.

Stone, M. (1981) *The Education of the Black Child: The Myth of Multi-cultural Education*, London: Fontana.

Stone, M. (1985) *The Education of the Black Child: The Myth of Multi-cultural Education*, 2nd edn, London: Fontana.

Stonequist, E. V. (1937) *The Marginal Man: A Study in Personality and Culture Conflict*, New York: Charles Sribner's Sons.

Stopes-Roe, M. and Cochrane, R. (1990) *Citizens of this Country: The Asian–British*, Clevedon: Multilingual Matters.

Stubbs, P. (1988) 'The reproduction of racism in state social work', unpublished PhD thesis, University of Bath.

Sue, D. W. and Sue, D. (1981) *Counselling the Culturally Different*, New York: Wiley & Sons.

Sue, D. W. and Sue, D. (1990) *Counselling the Culturally Different*, 2nd edn, New York: Wiley & Sons.

Sue, D. W. and Sue, D. (1999) *Counseling the Culturally Different: Theory and Practice*, 3rd edn, New York: Wiley & Sons.

Sue, D. W. and Sue, D. (2003) *Counseling the Culturally Different: Theory and Practice*, 4th edn, New York: Wiley & Sons.

Sue, S. (1978) 'Ethnic minority research: trends and directions', paper presented at *National Conference on Minority Group Alcohol, Drug Abuse and Mental Health Issues*, Denver.

Sue, D. W. (2006) *Multicultural Social Work Practice*, Hoboken, NJ: Wiley & Sons.

Sue, S. and Wagner, N. (eds.) (1973) *Asian Americans: Psychological Perspectives*, Palo Alto, CA: Science and Behaviour Books.

Swann, M. (1985) *Education for All: Final Report of the Committee of Inquiry into the Education of Children from Ethnic Minority Groups*, Cmnd 9453, London: HMSO.

Tajfel, H. (1981) *Human Groups and Social Categories: Studies in Social Psychology*, Cambridge: Cambridge University Press.

Tajfel, H. (1982) 'Social psychology of inter-group relations', *Annual Review of Psychology*, 33: 1–39.

Taylor, J. (1976) 'Psychosocial development among Black children and youth: a re-examination', *American Journal of Orthopsychiatry*, 46: 4–19.

Taylor, M. and Hegarty, S. (1986) *Between Two Cultures*, Windsor: NFER.

Terman, L. (1916) *The Measurement of Intelligence*, Cambridge, MA: Riverside Press.

Terrel, F. and Terrell, S. (1984) 'Race of Counselor, Client Sex, Cultural Mistrust Level, and Premature Termination from Counseling among Black Clients', *Journal of Counseling Psychology*, 31, 3: 371–5.

Tewfik, G. I. and Okasha, A. (1965) 'Psychosis and immigration', *Postgraduate Medical Journal*, 41: 603–12.

Thoburn, J., Norford, L. and Rashid, S. P. (2000) *Permanent Family Placement for Children of Minority Ethnic Origin*, London: Jessica Kinsley Publishers.

Thomas, A. and Sillen, S. (1972) *Racism and Psychiatry*, Secaucus, NJ: The Citadel Press.

Thomas, A. and Sillen, S. (1974) 'The significance of the e(thnocentrism) factor in mental health', *Journal of Social Issues*, 2: 60–9.

Thomas, C. S. and Comer, J. P. (1973) 'Racism and mental health services', in C. V. Willie, B. M. Kramer and B. S. Brown (eds.) *Racism in Mental Health*, Pittsburgh: University of Pittsburgh.

Thomas, C. W. (1971) *Boys No More*, Beverly Hills, CA: Glencoe Press.

Thomas, C. W. and Thomas, S. W. (1971) 'Blackness is a tonic', in C. W. Thomas, *Boys No More*, Beverly Hills, CA: Glencoe Press.

Thompson, C. P., Anderson, L. P. and Bakeman, R. A. (2000) 'Effects of racial socialization and racial identity on acculturative stress in African American college students', *Cultural Diversity and Ethnic Minority Psychology*, 6, 2: 196–210.

Thompson, N. (2001) *Anti-discriminatory Practice*, 3rd edn, Basingstoke: Macmillan.

Thorndike, E. L. (1940) *Human Nature and the Social Order*, New York: Macmillan.

Thorndike, E. L. (1968) 'Review of R. Rosenthal and L. Jacobson, Pygmalion in the Classroom', *American Educational Research Journal*, 5: 708–11.

Thornton, M. C., Chatters, L. M., Taylor, R. J. and Allen, W. R. (1990) 'Sociodemographic and environmental correlates of racial socialization by Black parents', *Child Development*, 61: 401–9.

Tizard, B. and Phoenix, A. (1989) 'Black identity and transracial adoption', *New Community*, 15, 3: 427–38.

Tizard, B. and Phoenix, A. (1993) *Black, White or Mixed Race: Race and Racism in the Lives of Young People of Mixed Parentage*, London: Routledge.

Tizard, B. and Phoenix, A. (2003) *Black, White or Mixed Race: Race and Racism in the Lives of Young People of Mixed Parentage*, 2nd edn, London: Routledge.

Toliver, S.D. (1998) *Black Families in Corporate America*, London: Sage Publications.

Tomlinson, S. (1983) *Ethnic Minorities in British Schools: a Review of the Literature, 1960–1982*, Aldershot: Gower.

Tomlinson, S. (1991) 'Ethnicity and educational attainment in England: an overview', *Anthropology and Education Quarterly*, 22: 121–39.

Tomlinson, S. (1992) 'Disadvantaging the disadvantaged: Bangladeshis and education in Tower Hamlets', *British Journal of Sociology of Education*, 13, 4: 437–46.

Tomlinson, S. (2005) 'Race, Ethnicity and Education Under New Labour', *Oxford Review of Education*, 31, 1: 153–71.

Treacher, A. and Katz, I. (eds.) (2000) *The Dynamics of Adoption*, London: Jessica Kingsley.

Triandis, H. C. and Brislin, R. W. (1984) 'Cross-cultural psychology', *American Psychologist*, 39, 9: 1006–16.

Trimble, J. E., Helms, J. E. and Root, M. P. P. (2003). 'Social and psychological perspectives in ethnic and racial identity', in G. Bernal, J. Trimble, and F. Leong (eds.) *Handbook of Racial and Ethnic Minority Psychology, Part III, Social and Developmental Process*, Thousand Oaks, CA: Sage Publications.

Triseliotis, J. (ed.) (1972) *Social Work with Coloured Immigrants and their Families*, London: Institute of Race Relations/Oxford University Press.

Troyna, B. (1984) 'Fact or artefact? The "educational underachievement" of Black pupils', *British Journal of Sociology of Education*, 5, 2: 153–66.

Troyna, B. and Williams, J. (1986) *Racism, Education and the State*, Beckenham: Croom Helm.

Tsui, P. (1997) 'The dynamics of cultural and power relations in group therapy', in E. Lee (ed.) *Working with Asian Americans: A guide for clinicians*, New York: Haworth Press.

Tsui, P. and Schultz, G. L. (1988) 'Ethnic factors in group process: cultural dynamics in multi-ethnic group therapy groups', *American Journal of Orthopsychiatry Bulletin*, 58, 1: 136–42.

Tuckwell, G (2002) *Racial Identity, White Counsellors and Therapists*, Buckingham: Open University Press.

Tyson, G. A. (1985) 'Children's racial attitudes: a review', unpublished Human Science Research Council report, Pretoria.

Uba, L. (1994) *Asian Americans: Personality Patterns, Identity and Mental Health*, New York: Guilford Press.

Uhlenberg, J. and Brown, K. M. (2002) 'Racial Gap in Teachers' Perceptions of the Achievement Gap', *Education and Urban Society*, 34, 4: 493–530.

Valentine, C. A. (1971) 'Deficit, difference, and bicultural models of Afro-American behavior', *Harvard Educational Review*, 41, 2: 137–57.

Vandiver, B. J, (2001) 'Psychological nigrescence revisited: Introduction and overview', *Journal of Multicultural Counseling and Development*, 29: 165–73.

Vaughan, G. M. (1964) 'The development of ethnic attitudes in New Zealand school children', *Genetic Psychology Monographs*, 70: 135–75.

Verma, G. K. with Ashworth, B. (1986) *Ethnicity and Educational Achievement in British Schools*, London: Macmillan.

Verma, G. K. and Pumfrey, P. (eds.) (1988) *Educational Attainments: Issues and Outcomes in Multicultural Education*, London: Falmer Press.

Vontress, C. E. (1971) 'Racial differences: impediments to rapport', *Journal of Counseling Psychology*, 18: 7–13.

Ward, C. (1996) 'Acculturation', in D. Landis and R. Bhagat (eds.) *Handbook of Intercultural Training*, 2nd edn, Thousand Oaks, CA: Sage Publications.

Watson, D. M. (1970) *Proxemic Behaviours: A Cross-Cultural Study*, The Hague: Mouton.

Watt, D., Sheriffe, G. and Majors, R. (1999) *Mentoring Black Male Pupils*, unpublished manuscript, City College, Manchester.

Weaver, D. (1982) 'Empowering treatment skills for helping black families', *Social Casework*, 63: 100–5.

Webb-Johnson, A. (1991) *A Cry for Change: An Asian Perspective on Developing Quality Mental Health Care*, London: Confederation of Indian Organisations.

Weitz, S. (1972) 'Attitude, voice, and behaviour: a repressed effect model of interracial behaviour', *Journal of Personality and Social Psychology*, 24: 14–21.

Westwood, S. and Bhachu, P. (1988) 'Images and Realities', *New Society*, 6 May.

Whaley, A. L. (2001) 'Cultural Mistrust and Mental Health Services for African Americans', *The Counseling Psychologist*, 29, 4: 513–31.

White, J. (1970) 'Toward a black psychology', *Ebony*, 25, 11: 44–52.

White, J. and Cones, J. (1999) *Black Men Emerging*, New York: Routledge.

White, J. L. (1972) 'Toward a black psychology', in R. L. Jones (ed.) *Black Psychology*, New York: Harper & Row.

White, J. L. (1980) 'Toward a black psychology', in R. L. Jones (ed.) *Black Psychology*, 2nd edn, New York: Harper & Row.

White, J. L. (1984) *The Psychology of Blacks: An Afro-American Perspective*, Englewood Cliffs, NJ: Prentice-Hall.

White, J. L. (1991) 'Toward a black psychology', in R. L. Jones (ed.) *Black Psychology*, 3rd edn, Berkeley, CA: Cobb & Henry.

White, J. L. (2004) 'Toward a Black Psychology', in R. L. Jones (ed.) *Black Psychology*, 4th edn, New York: Harper & Row.

White, J. L. and Johnson, A. J. (1972) 'Awareness, pride and identity: a positive educational strategy for black youth', in R. Jones (ed.) *Black Psychology*, New York: Harper & Row.

Wijeyesinghe, C. L. and Jackson, B. W. (2001) *New Perspectives on Racial Identity Development: A theoretical and practical anthology*, New York: New York University Press.

Wilkinson, D. (1974) 'Racial socialization through children's toys: a socio-historical examination', *Journal of Black Studies*, 5: 96–109.

Wilkinson, D. (1980) 'Play objects as tools of propaganda: characterizations of the African-American male', *Journal of Black Psychology*, 7, 1: 1–16.

Williams, D. R. (2003) 'The health of men: Structured inequalities and opportunities', *American Journal of Public Health*, 93, 5: 725–31.

Williams, I. J. (1975) 'An investigation of the developmental stages of Black consciousness', PhD thesis, University of Cincinnati. Dissertation Abstracts International 36, 5B: 2488–9.

Williams, R. (1972) 'Abuses and misuses in testing black children', in R. L. Jones (ed.) *Black Psychology*, New York: Harper & Row.

Williams, R. L. (1975) 'The BITCH-100: a culture-specific test', *Journal of Afro-American Issues*, 3, 103–14.

Williams, R. L. (1978) *Black Psychology: Compelling Issues and Views*, Washington, DC: Associated Publishers.

Williams, R. L. (1981) *The Collective Black Mind: An Afro-centric Theory of Black Personality*, St. Louis, MO: Williams.

Williams, R. L. and Mitchell, H. (1981) 'The testing game', in R. Jones (ed.) *Black Psychology*, 2nd edn, New York: Harper & Row.

Williams, R. A., Williams, R. L. and Mitchell, H. (2004) 'The testing game', in R. Jones (ed.) *Black Psychology*, 4th edn, New York: Harper & Row.

Willie, C. V. (1970) *The Family Life of Black People*, Columbus, OH: Charles E.Merrill.

Willie, C. V. (1982) *A New Look at Black Families*, 2nd edn, Bayside, NY: General Hall.

Willie, C. V., Kramer, M. and Brown, B. S. (eds.) (1973) *Racism and Mental Health*, Pittsburgh, PA: University of Pittsburgh Press.

Willis, F. N. (1966) 'Initial speaking distance as a function of the speakers' relationship', *Psychonomic Science*, 5: 221–2.

Willis, F. N. and Hoffman, G. E. (1975) 'Development of tactile patterns in relationship to age, sex and race', *Development Psychology*, 11: 866.

Willis, F., Reeves, D. and Buchanan, D. (1976) 'Interpersonal touch in high school relative to sex and race', *Perceptual and Motor Skills*, 43: 843–7.

Wilson, A. (1978) *The Developmental Psychology of the Black Child*, New York: Africana Research Publications.

Wilson, A. (1981) 'The psychological development of the black child', *Black Books Bulletin*, 7, 2: 8–14.

Wilson, A. (1987) *Mixed Race Children: A Study of Identity*, London: Allen Unwin.

Wilson, A. (1992) *Awakening the Natural Genius of Black Children*, New York: Afrikan World Infosystems.

Winkel, F. W. and Vrij, A. (1990) 'Interaction and impression formation in a cross-cultural dyad: frequency and meaning of culturally determined gaze behaviour in a police interview setting', *Social Behaviour*, 5: 335–50.

Wong, A. (1986) 'Creole as a language of power and solidarity', in D. Sutcliffe and A. Wong (eds.) *The Language of the Black Experience*, Oxford: Basil Blackwell.

Word, C. O., Zanna, M. P. and Cooper, J. (1974) 'The non-verbal mediation of self-fulfilling prophecies in interracial interaction', *Journal of Experimental Social Psychology*, 10: 109–20.

Wrench, J. and Hassan, E. (1996) *Ambition and Marginalisation: A Qualitative Study of Underachieving Young Men of Afro-Caribbean Origin*, London: DfEE.

Wright, C. (1986) 'School processes: an ethnographic study', in J. Eggleston, D. Dunn, and M. Anjali (eds.) *Education for Some: The Educational and Vocational Experiences of 15–18-year-old Members of Minority Ethnic Groups*, Stoke-on-Trent: Trentham Books.

Wylie, R. (1978) *The Self-Concept, Vol. 2, Theory and Research on Selected Topics*, revised edition, Lincoln, NA: University of Nebraska Press.

Yalom, I. D. (1975) *The Theory and Practice of Group Psychotherapy*, New York: Basic Books.

Yalom, I. D. (1985) *The Theory and Practice of Group Psychotherapy*, 3rd edn, New York: Basic Books.

Yalom. I. D. (2005) *The Theory and Practice of Group Psychotherapy*, 5th edn, New York: Basic Books.

Yee, A. H., Fairchild, H. H., Weizmann, F. and Wyatt, G.E. (1993) 'Addressing psychology's problem with race', *American Psychologist*, 48, 1132–40.

Yeh, C. J. and Huang, K. (1996) 'The collectivistic nature of ehtnic identity development among Asian American college students', *Adolescence*, 31: 645–61.

Yelloly, M. A. (1980, 1990) *Social Work Theory and Psychoanalysis*, London: Van Nostrand Reinhold.

Zeitlin, H. (2002) 'Adoption of children from minority groups', in K. N. Dwivedi (ed.) *Meeting the Needs of Ethnic Minority Children*, London: Jessica Kingsley Publishers.

Subject Index

Author index